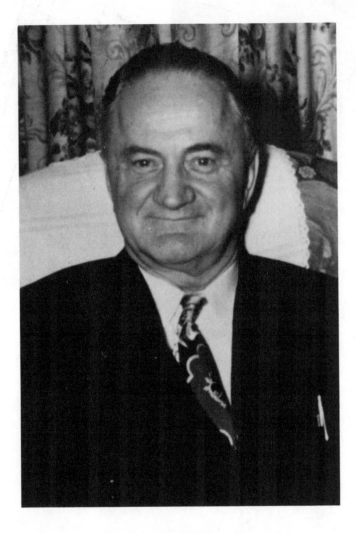

DR. RANDOLPH STONE AT AGE 60.

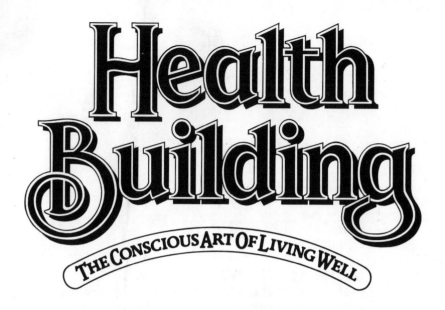

Health Building

The Conscious Art Of Living Well

DR. RANDOLPH STONE, D.O., D.C.

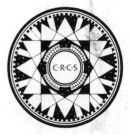

CRCS PUBLICATIONS
P.O. Box 20850
Reno, NV 89515
U.S.A.

Library of Congress Cataloging in Publication Data

Stone, Randolph, 1890-1981
  Health building.

  Includes bibliographical references.
  1. Health. 2. Vitality. 3. Holistic medicine.
4. Nutrition. 5. Exercise. I. Title.
RA776.S868 1985   613   84-71547
ISBN 0-916360-23-7 (pbk.)

This book includes revised and expanded editions of the author's previously published booklets *Health Building, A Purifying Diet, Easy Stretching Postures,* and various other articles and writings.

INTERNATIONAL STANDARD BOOK NUMBER: 0-916360-23-7
LIBRARY OF CONGRESS CATALOG CARD NUMBER: 84-71547
Published simultaneously in the United States and Canada by:
CRCS Publications
Distributed in the United States and internationally by
CRCS Publications
(Write for current list of worldwide distributors.)
Cover Design: Image & lettering both by Rebecca Wilson

NOTE FOR HEALTH PRACTITIONERS: Quantity discounts on this book are available to health practitioners, teachers, health centers & retreats, etc. Write CRCS Publications for information stating quantity desired.

Contents

PART II: EASY STRETCHING POSTURES FOR VITALITY & BEAUTY

Other Books by Author
Information on Polarity Therapy Associations

Publisher's Note

CRCS Publications is proud to publish the first popular trade editions of Dr. Randolph Stone's work. This volume comprises all of Dr. Stone's writings that were specifically intended for his patients and which therefore are written in an informal, conversational style. Originally published as small self-help manuals to encourage people to take an energetic part in rebuilding their health, the material in this volume is an integral part of Dr. Stone's approach to health. In his practice, he used the dietary, exercise, and mental principles described herein along with Polarity Therapy energy balancing treatments and sometimes other physical therapies.

For Dr. Stone, health is a positive state of well-being, not just the absence of obvious disease. It is a state of being that one can *build* through effort, discipline, responsibility, and persistence. And that state of well-being is achieved by the stimulation and balancing of the life energies which flow in definite patterns and finer energy fields throughout the human constitution. Seeing and working with the human being as a complex coordination of subtle energy fields was the foundation of all Dr. Stone's work and the secret of his remarkable successes with many "hopeless cases." (As he got older, he specialized more and more in difficult cases whom other doctors had failed to help.)

In addition to diet and exercises, Dr. Stone discusses the spiritual and psychological dimensions of life and their relation to health and wholeness. Those dimensions of being are also an integral part of his therapeutic perspective and cannot be separated from the more commonplace subjects of diet and exercise. For Dr. Stone, all of the dimensions of a human being are important, and the striking simplicity and clarity of his wholistic vision of life was a rare gift that powerfully affected many people who came into contact with him.

For the modern mind, the unpretentious simplicity of some of his views might be difficult to accept, so accustomed are we to detailed analysis and endless complexity. It has to be acknowledged that Dr. Stone spoke and wrote in an inspired, stream-of-consciousness style, and he was in fact a uniquely effective communicator of subtle truths.* The reader encountering Dr. Stone for the first time must relax his or her critical mind somewhat and be truly open to the flow of thought and vision of life that Dr. Stone is expressing in order to receive the maximum benefit and understanding from his writings. Dr. Stone was not interested in impressing academics but in *communicating* to the masses a powerful, holistic truth that he felt was being almost completely neglected in the modern world and in the healing arts.

It would be accurate to say that Dr. Stone's "all-at-onceness" quality of perception is reflected in his writing style. Therefore, we did not want to edit it too much to make it sound like a dry academic treatise or a journalistic report. The proof of his ideas is in the results, and many individuals who have followed his health principles have benefited greatly and have found them powerfully effective. As Dr. Stone writes,

> If you will follow the entire routine strictly, without consulting your own opinions, habits and appetites, you will notice improvements that will astonish you. If you want to follow your own inclinations or habits, why consult a doctor? (page 92)

The unity of Dr. Stone's life-vision is nowhere more evident than in his wide-ranging references to many different religious, occult, spiritual, therapeutic, and cultural images and terms. This was quite natural for him since he was a life-long truthseeker whose diversity of interests knew no bounds. He draws on many Western and Eastern traditions to present a remarkably integrated view of human functioning, and he found that many ancient systems (including Yoga, Ayurvedic medicine, Astrology, and the Kaballah) described the fields of energy which sustain the human body. Those interested in pursuing his research in more detail than this book provides should read his collected works on the energy-balancing art and science that he called "Polarity Therapy".†

---

*Many of the quotations at the beginning of chapters are taken from Dr. Stone's lectures and workshops. Unless otherwise identified, all the other quotations are excerpted from his published writings or notebooks.

†Those wishing to learn the practice and techniques of Polarity Therapy should also contact a qualified Polarity Therapy teacher. See the back of this volume for the addresses of Polarity Therapy Associations that can refer you to teachers and practitioners.

Finally, it must be pointed out that this book does not attempt to diagnose or treat specific illnesses. It is advisable to seek professional advice or to consult your physician in every case where you are in doubt about your health, particularly when you have persistent pain or any other continuous symptom. The publisher of this book takes no responsibility for the reader's health or use or misuse of the information contained herein.

Acknowledgements

The publisher wishes to thank Jim Feil for editorial help, Dr. James Said for providing quotations from Dr. Stone's seminars, Dr. Robert K. Hall for one of the photos and for writing the foreword, and Dr. Stone's niece Louise Hilger for providing photos and encouragement.

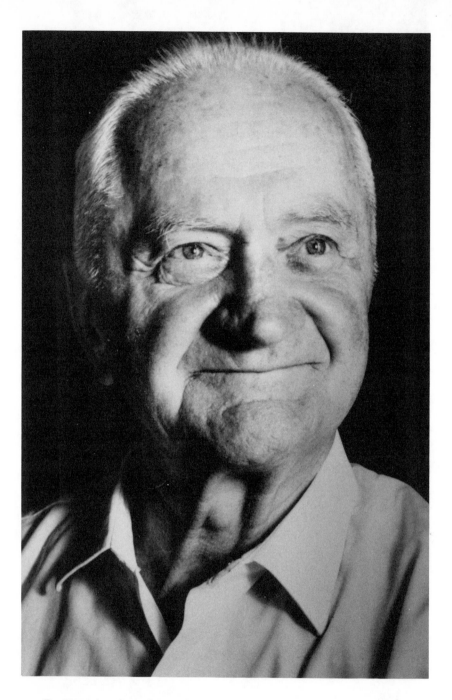

Dr. Stone in a formal portrait taken in India when he was in his eighties.

Foreword

Were he alive today, Randolph Stone would be delighted that his books are finally being professionally published. His work was for him second in importance only to his Spiritual Master. He was a teacher who taught constantly. Every conversation I ever had with him contained some new revelation in his thinking about energy and the human organism. His teaching still lives through hundreds of his students, who are doing his work all over the world. He would be happy to know that.

In 1948 he published his first book himself. It was called *The New Energy Concept Of The Healing Art.** In 1953 he published *The Wireless Anatomy Of Man*, containing many hand-drawn charts "which illustrate the fields of potential wireless energy currents in the human body." Later he wrote, "these fields became the fulcrum for moving and releasing stagnant wireless currents in the body by means of polarity contacts and skillful manipulation *based upon energy flow*, unlike the accepted view which deals with the nervous system as [the only] conductor." (Unpublished paper entitled *Energy— A New Viewpoint Discovered For The Healing Art*, June 25, 1957.) In 1954, he published a new text called *Polarity Therapy* and also his small book for the lay public called *Easy Stretching Postures For Vitality and Beauty*. (He certainly knew what would appeal to the lay public!)

In 1957 he wrote, "But the [energy concept applied to the healing arts] is so new to the average person's thinking pattern that it takes time to penetrate and to make a change in the basic thinking and viewpoint." He was very excited that an "energetic group of drugless doctors in Seattle" who had studied his books and taken his courses had formed an interesting new center called "The National Polarity Therapy Association." Now almost thirty years later, there are Polarity Therapy Centers across the entire United States.

---

*Beginning with the second revised, expanded edition of this book, it was retitled *Energy: The Vital Polarity in the Healing Art*.

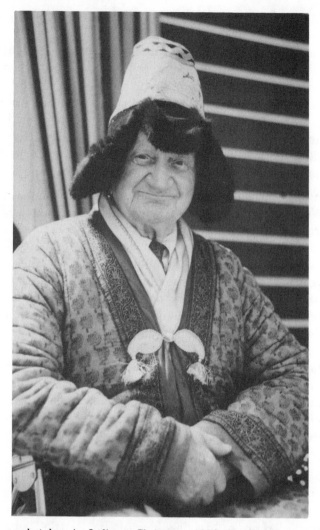

Photograph taken in India at Christmas, 1973. Dr. Stone wrote of this outfit on the photo: "The robes were specially made to order by tailors of the old Rajahs in Jaipur. They are so dignified and comfortably warm for meditation in this cold weather here this year. The cap is also a specially designed royal gift to me. . . . It is of heavy fur with a gold top and trimmings. It comes from Kathmandu in Nepal on the Chinese border. This is an unusual combination I could not show or wear anywhere else. . . . It is an appropriate birthday present for me at 84 years next month." (Photo courtesy of Dr. Robert K. Hall.)

What was this idea, so revolutionary that Dr. Stone was amazed whenever a physician became interested in his work? What was so difficult about what he taught that he fully expected *not* to be understood?

He taught what is today being called the new paradigm, the "New Physics." He taught that the human flesh we identify as our own bodies is not, in fact, a solid thing, but a system of coordinated energy patterns that are generally in movement. It was his discovery that sickness results from specific inhibitions in the flow of this energy. And he spent fifty or more years developing manual methods of healing human malfunctioning, by learning to restore natural movement of the energy fields. He also was a living model of the effectiveness of his own methods. He taught them and demonstrated their truth. He used his own discoveries in his daily life, and his energetic appearance and numinous vitality were as much proof of what he taught as were the many people whose lives were immediately enriched by the touch of his hands. He was a divinely inspired healer and he was a pioneer physician.

I once asked him where his information about energy channels originated. He laughed and told me that he "burned the midnight oil." I knew that, by this, he referred to his meditation practice. He learned about the movement of energy and its "step-down" into matter "by studying himself." Such is the path of genius when not contaminated by the ego's harping.

There was a special insistent quality about his touch. When he directed attention to someone's suffering body, a demand was transmitted from his hands to the other's awareness. It was a call to life, an insistence on becoming conscious. Many times I watched resistant flesh begin to release its contraction and vibrate under his hands. Then he would laugh and proclaim the simplicity of the whole procedure. "It's just energy blocks in the connective tissue," he would exclaim, "probably poor digestion, yes, we only need to help it along a little *here!*" And his patient would be wide-eyed with astonishment at the cascade of feelings that were being catalyzed by this man's

stubby thumbs. He was a healer whose hands probed and ex-
plored. Inevitably they sought out the place where the soul
was hiding, refusing to expand or struggling to open. It was
there, in that hidden place, that Dr. Stone did his wonderful
work.

Now he has been gone from us for quite some time. More
conventional scientists are just beginning to walk along path-
ways that he long ago charted. Those of us who were fortunate
enough to have stood with him and received his transmission
were imprinted indelibly by his enthusiastic wisdom. It seems
proper that we applaud the new editions of his written work
that are being published by CRCS Publications. Often in these
inspired texts, the very spirit of our old teacher speaks. He
looks out at us again from behind a sentence stuffed with
meaning, and points to the truth of God's love, found in the
human body, the temple more real than all the world's cathe-
drals. Randolph Stone knew that. He knew that the body is as
much the manifestation of God's presence as is Holy Scripture.
He saw himself as a janitor of the temple, one who knew how
to sweep out the dust and prepare the rooms for the coming of
light. I am honored to invite you to study what the old janitor
wrote about his work. His writings have accumulated historical
value now, but there is no decrease in their power to transmit
revolutionary ideas. Although the knowledge they reveal is
ancient, Dr. Stone managed to preserve and renew for us the
excitement, the inspiration that has always accompanied the
discovery of truth still alive, even in a darkened world.

Robert K. Hall, M.D.
Tomales, California
January, 1985
Lomi School

Part I

Health Building

Introduction

Health Consciousness:
The Essential Unity of Body,
Mind & Soul as the Key to Well-Being

*"The mind creates multiplicity everywhere to
cover the simplicity in nature."*

Health is not merely of the body. It is the natural expression of the body, mind and soul when they are in rhythm with the One Life. True health is the harmony of life within us, consisting of peace of mind, happiness and well-being. It is not merely a question of physical fitness, but is rather a result of the soul finding free expression through the mind and body of that individual. Such a person radiates peace and happiness, and everyone in his presence automatically feels happy and contented.

If we really want health, we must be willing to work for it, the same as we do for wealth, education or any other accomplishment in life. And those who seek health, truth and love will find it, if they devote themselves to it with zest and a purpose that never waivers. We become that which we contemplate. Negative thoughts and fears make grooves in the mind as negative energy waves of despondency and hopelessness. We cannot think negative thoughts and reap positive results, and therefore we must assert the positive, and maintain a positive pattern of thinking and acting as our ideal.

At the very core of the search for true health lies the essential question of what life is for. What is our personal goal, in terms of the use we make of this body and mind—and what is the purpose of the divine gift of this human life? Merely having no physical pain does not always mean a happy condition of mind. We are entitled to more and have a greater purpose for being in this world. Each one of us is seeking the inner happiness that comes not from outward accomplishments, but from the harmony of our inner being. What is life for, if it is not to make an effort to achieve a higher realization of consciousness? A realization of the soul, which gives us the uplift associated with the best of physical and mental health, and raises us far beyond the reach of the pain and anxiety caused by emotional, mental or physical dis-ease.

The soul functions in the body as conscious awareness, through the mind, the emotions, the senses and the electromagnetic sound and light waves. If we do not discipline our negative qualities of mind and emotion, we can never escape from ill health, in one form or another. Having experienced ill health and its pains, let us be determined to combat the intrusion of physical ailments, negative emotions and thoughts into this body-temple, by constant efforts to tune in to our higher consciousness and its healing powers.

"As we think, so we are." If we want health, we must learn to govern and direct our energies from the center outward, as expressions of life and motion, with a reverent attitude toward all life. We cannot kill for the sake of our palate without it having a profoundly destructive effect on our mental health, which in turn directly influences our physical fitness. Mentally, we have to inculcate in ourselves an approach which treats all life as the sacred gift of the Creator, and we as its steward. As a natural corollary, the ideal diet will consist of vegetables, fruits, nuts, seeds, grains, milk and milk products. These foods form a wholesome, balanced diet, which not only nourishes the body, but also appreciably lessens both emotional and mental tensions.

Besides such physical reactions as the toxins produced in our body when we eat the flesh of slaughtered animals, fish and fowl, there is also the factor of karma—that we inevitably reap what we have sown. We are responsible for all our actions, past and present, and experience the consequences in our physical, mental and emotional state of health. Hence, we are well advised to eat for health, by sowing the seeds of life, rather than sowing the seeds of future suffering through heedlessly abusing life each day.

If we form the habit of daily eating and drinking only for health—physical, mental and spiritual—we will find a growing sense of well-being, accompanied by the energy and happiness that come when one is no longer bound by cravings and appetites. We should not merely live to eat, blindly obeying our sense of taste, regardless of the consequences to ourselves and others; but we must strive to eat to live, in order to find peace within ourselves and be a source of love and happiness for all beings around us. We can rebuild and mold our body daily, psychologically and physically, while we avoid enervation through mental or physical excesses of any kind.

Each person should take enough time and interest to study his problem so that he or she can live intelligently and assist nature in tuning the body and mind into its abounding rhythm and beauty. To understand life, we must be in tune with it.

Those who are destined to look for true health will find it.

> *When Life and Love become our interest sublime,*
> *We do not need a personal self to shine.*

Life's own radiance exceeds all when we truly forget self and its limitations and sufferings, by being lost in Love and Life as the only jewel of Reality worth living for.

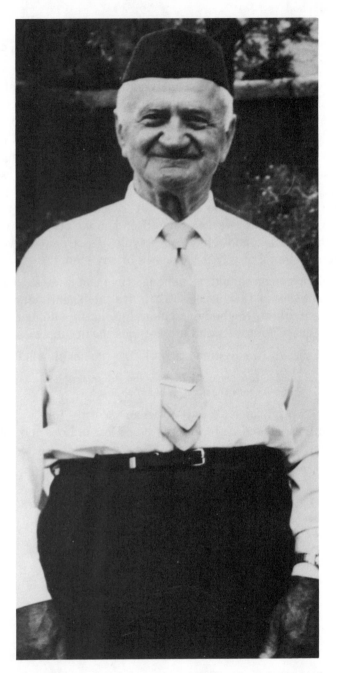

Dr. Stone in India during the 1970's, where he treated
hundreds of patients at a free clinic over a period of years
and where he encountered a wide variety of ailments and
especially difficult cases.

1

The Direct Approach to Healing: The Life Energy

"It is only the Energy in Matter that makes matter seem alive. When this energy escapes, only the shell is left. . . . A cure constitutes reaching the life current within and reestablishing the free flow of its energy."

When we are ill and have pains, we think that it is the body which hurts and is sick, when in reality it is the life-breaths or Prana Currents* in the body (which operate it and sustain it) which are out of balance and coordination in their polarity function of attraction and repulsion. This negative and positive action throughout the system is the factor which makes each cell contract and expand in its processes of life: to take in nourishment—of solids, liquids, gases, and warmth, or energy— use it and discard the waste products and gases, and radiate the heat (or caloric) energy for use and distribution.

This seems a new idea or concept, because we approach and explain it from the modern base of energy radiation, conduction and absorption, like electronic engineers would in their atomic research. This energy approach is prior to chemistry and mechanics. Energy in its threefold action of positive (+), negative (-), and neuter (0) polarity is prior to chemistry, which deals with particles of matter and their chemical affinity—or antipathy—which can result in new combinations or in an explosion of gases.

---

*Prana currents: In the Hindu tradition, *Prana* is a type of stored or radiant energy considered to be the life essence in all living forms.

We are still overly fascinated with the mechanical, chemical, and bacteriological aspects of matter in all our research in the healing arts, because we have lost the art of the direct approach through the life energy itself. All our scientific research is external to us—it is directed only by intellect, highly technical, and foreign to the oneness of the life process and its finer essences, by which we live and breathe and have our being. That is why we lack life in its full expression.

The energy approach through sound and light waves and electromagnetic tension fields has not yet been conceived or put into practice in the research on health and disease. It has been known locally but was lost again because matter is too great an illusion. It is through the electromagnetic energy tension fields that the sensory and motor energies in the body operate and function as secretion, and as the contraction and relaxation of muscle cells which produce motion.

The location of this energy is in the core of the brain and the spinal cord, where it exists as a highly vibrating intense etheric essence, of a neuter polarity as a molecular energy, which is the key to the entire structure and function of the body. This constitutes the Wireless Anatomy of Man as a molecular field of energy substance and its radiation or aura. Direct conduction of this wireless molecular essence is through the brain and its cortex as well as the meninges and its interspaces, which become the highly charged electromagnetic fields of positive and negative polarity, expressed in the right and left life breath through the two nostrils. This, in essence, is the picture of the NEW ENERGY CONCEPT OF THE HEALING ART* through electromagnetic polarity fields of expansion and contraction.

The body itself has no sensation, as it is matter. But these energy currents which permeate and run it are living messengers

---

*This book by Dr. Stone, now revised and entitled *Energy: The Vital Polarity in the Healing Art,* is included in the collected works of Dr. Stone, available from CRCS Publications.

to the life within at its core, and to the consciousness which is the Soul. All pain is but an obstruction to this energy flow, in its molecular and conducted fields through the nerves which act as wires for direct and specific energy impulses from a switch area in the brain to a point of function in the body.

The cerebrospinal fluid is the liquid medium for this life energy radiation, expansion and contraction. Where this is present, there is life and healing with normal function. Where this primary and essential life force is not acting in the body, there is obstruction, spasm, or stagnation and pain, like gears which clash instead of meshing in their operation.

This new approach to the healing art should release the mind of the excessive fear of disease and germs, which can be a great depressing factor and stand in the way of normal recovery. Are germs more potent than the life within, the God-given heritage? Life is a river of energy which must flow to keep clear and sweet in its function through all the organisms of life's expression. Only when life's currents are obstructed and become stagnant does fermentation of waste in the tissues cause decay and germs. Their origin is in decomposition.

Life is a centrifugal energy in its operation, which rules supreme where it acts and functions. So the primary effort of the healing art should be to get life to flow through stagnant and obstructed areas and tissues of the body which cause pain. That is the natural way, from the inside out and from the top down, as the centrifugal force operates. But all effort should be to help to establish this normal energy flow and not merely to suppress symptoms of elimination, by pain-killing suppressant drugs. A cure constitutes reaching the life current within and re-establishing a free flow of its energy currents. Anything short of this is but a relief measure.

Now we come to the psychological aspects of disease, where the emotions and mind are great factors. What a patient fears, believes or thinks affects his health and can create energy blocks in the emotional field as well as in the mind pattern energy which governs the electromagnetic fields in their essence energy and sets the patterns for the positive and negative current flow.

The awareness of life as energy currents, and their regulation toward normal flow, is the key to the natural art of health-building: regulating the food and drink, the emotions and the mind—all to the pattern of nature and its rational rhythm and keynote.

2

Health-Building Ideas

*This house of clay in which we stay
And where we play and also pray,
Is our temple and our fort, for life's sport,
Built from mind and feeling patterns
    long and short.*

*We are what we eat and drink
What we feel and what we think.
"Man does not live by bread alone."
Mind patterns rule our life.*

Sound and Light Waves

Life is the expression of love in sound waves and energy
currents, throughout the creation and in man. Love is light,
which crystalizes as beauty in the spectrum, becomes color
and gases as it is reduced in speed of vibration, and also forms
the beautiful colors in the buds, the flowers, and the fruits. It
precipitates as the delicate pink color of the lacework of tissues
in the human form. Everywhere is the expression of love and
beauty as art and design patterns. Concentrated waves form
electromagnetic fields, build the cells and govern them by
attraction and repulsion. The three gunas* are everywhere the
attributes of matter and motion, as positive (+), negative (-),
and neuter (0). Everywhere is life in motion and in sound
effects, such as speech, the songs of birds, and the lowing of
beasts or their roar of life's expression. There is music everywhere as plus and minus tones, without and within, if we can

---

*Gunas: The universal principles governing all motion. In his advanced
texts, Dr. Stone uses the gunas as a mode of categorizing various types
of therapeutic interventions.

but hear it and see it in love and understanding of the Creator's Grace and Being.

"Life is one." "The Lord our God is One."

He is the essence of all life and beauty everywhere. With this keynote of understanding, life flows like a river of natural expression and manifests as health.

Positive Mind Patterns

To have health, we must have it in mind as an ideal pattern and an objective to work for. We must lay out our days' work and habits in line with that blueprint of health and life— actively doing and being as we want to be. Then all will be a harmonious expression with a purpose in life, in love with the Creator and His wonderful creation.

He is in all there is as the one Essence, the One Life, the One Love, and the One Understanding of Truth. This keynote must be established as the positive mind pattern in the seeker of health, and by the positive attitude of daily realization and becoming in thought, in deeds, in actions and in feeling at one within oneself and with Nature outside.

Then these patterns will attract the positive particles of space energy and fill the patterns of cells and tissue formation with life's ions as we live, breathe and think in terms of love and life as our reality and heritage. We will become that which we contemplate.

Negative thoughts and fears attract negative ions to build into our mind space negative thought waves and negative energy waves, feelings of despondency and hopelessness. All this occurs because we have discarded the positive pattern of life as our ideal, our breath of life, and as our daily thinking on every subject and topic. We cannot think negative thoughts and reap positive results. We make the bed we lie on. We build the house we live in. If we really want health, we must be willing to work for it, the same as for wealth, education or other accomplishments in life. And those who seek health, truth or love shall find it if they devote themselves to it with zest and a purpose that never wavers in its course.

Life is a river; it is a road—a direction of energy waves and currents in our being that leads to more water of life, more space and tolerance and to higher pinnacles of love and understanding, through pleasure and pain, through success and failure, through trials and overcoming all our negative factors of thinking, doing and feeling, into a harmony of love and its fullness of expression through understanding and compassion.

Soulful Living

Health is not merely of the body, it is one in all. It is the natural expression of the Soul, of love, of life in rhythm with the One Life, its Source and supply house. Happiness is of the Soul, in love of oneness and unity, the reality of being. The body is an earthy Temple and has only the happiness in its fields which the thinker or artist in the body builds into it, by thinking designs and patterns of happiness and health. "As we think so we are." All our efforts must be toward health as a unit of accomplishment and life itself in daily habits of eating and drinking for health only. We must not merely obey our sense of taste or cravings and habits of the past. Life must have a definite purpose and meaning. It is a road that leads somewhere. Where is our guiding Star, and our Goal? What is life for, if it is not an effort to higher realization of consciousness or Soul growth and inner happiness? We can become that which we wish to be if we work for it.

Objectives and Life's Jewel

Possessions, position and condition are but means to an end, not the end in itself. We must use these wisely, or they will use us as slaves and servants to their design and pattern of more and more greed and exhaustion through frustration, enervation and bad health. If you wish to gain health and happiness, you must work for it and labor in its vineyard all hours, day and night, in thoughts and in deeds and hold fast to the One Idea—the Jewel of Life within you. Have you ever asked yourself, if I gain health, what will I do with it? What for? Have I learned my lesson of inharmony and mistakes by suffering and through illness? Be an artist and an architect of your own house, your temple, your body and your mind. Build and struggle, and don't expect anybody else to do it for you, so you can let your mind wander loose without direction or control. All life points to this one lesson—mind control through love and understanding. If this is not the objective in our life, why bother at all to look for health? Health and happiness do not depend on the body, but on the energies that run it, flow through it and animate it.

If we want health we must learn to govern and direct those energies from the center outward as normal expressions of life and motion, with a reverent attitude toward life's sacredness as the Creator's gift and we as its steward. We are held responsible for it and experience it by action and reaction. Life is but a kindergarten of experience. We learn by positive and negative actions and reactions, as cause and effect, which are life's lights and shadows.

If you are interested in your health, start to think on causes and effects, and you won't need to look for an escape mechanism or wonder pill or tranquilizers to do the work for you. We must learn to live life and feed the body wholesome natural foods with all the life elements in it, in their finer forms as enzymes, hormones, vitamins, and minerals, besides the bulk of proteins, starches, sweets and fats to nourish the grosser parts and serve as combustive material in the digestive process.

Health

Getting well is a road of labor and of love; it is won through effort; then we reach this ideal condition. If we set our hand to the plow of well-being, we cannot turn back without losing all that was gained. If we discard the blueprints of our new pattern of life, then the house will not be built and we remain in our shack and shackles of a ruined temple and its derelict appearance of disease.

Life does not tolerate disease. Then why should we? If we do not struggle with our negative qualities of mind and emotions like a fish caught in a net, we never can escape those loops and bonds. Having experienced ill health and its pains, let us be determined to understand its cause and change this effect and gain control of our fort of life. Why let negative intruders rule and wreck our temple? Disease is the negation and the lack of life. And negative thinking and attitudes invite it, and attract those ions as precipitated feeling and moods of suffering. Are we the master of our house, or not? Shall doubts or negative emotions and thoughts destroy the sacredness of our shrine of life within?

We either walk with Nature's energies and work with them by depending on the glorious life within and its radiant self, or we look for substitutes on the outside and become victims to sedatives and narcotics as a bad habit and weakness of life itself, because they depress life. Life must be king in our temple of being. Escape mechanisms are not worthy of life's purpose.

The Labyrinth of Life

The way out of this Labyrinth of Life is by going deeper within and becoming acquainted with life itself, its radiant glory, its energy rays and currents, and its ever-present helpfulness in need, if we seek it and depend upon it. It is the Creator's Hand that reaches down and lifts up the energy currents of our mind and feelings, through love and concentrated devotion at the core of life within our own sanctuary of being.

When Life and Love become our interest sublime,
We do not need a personal self to shine.

Life's own radiance exceeds all when we truly forget self and its limitations and sufferings, by being lost in Love and Life as the One Jewel of Reality worth living for.

3

Principles & Application

"Creation has an outward purpose for the body and an inward purpose for the soul. . . . The creation which we see with our material eyes, and only part of which we can comprehend, is but a very, very small part of the total Creation . . . it is but a speck of the Real Grand Total of the entire expanse of finer and still finer Substance and Vastness beyond the comprehension of the mind."

Digestion is a process of combustion of solids or liquids to extract their heat units as energy for motion and their chemistry for replacing worn-out particles in the body tissues. "Combustion is a rapid chemical union of light and heat; its by-products are CO_2 (carbon dioxide) and water (moisture)." Combustion in an engine and in our digestive system is similar—and very informative by comparison.

The fuel for an engine must be suitable for that type of engine and combustion chamber, whether it be a steam or gasoline engine. This is an important point in building health and maintaining it. Even wealthy men, like John D. Rockefeller who had a very poor digestive system all his life, by very careful selection and light eating of simple foods lived to a ripe old age. The Italian nobleman, Cornario, proved the same point. He lived to be 110 years old because he lived a simple life after he was told by doctors that he would die in his early youth because of his reckless habits.

A little thinking and attention applied to our own motor and its combustion proportions and quality would save us much ill health and suffering. On the process of digestion depends the maintenance of our body the same as the performance of the motor. Only with this exception: The body is a self-repairing machine with emotion and the mind as the finer energy spark plugs to ignite ambition and all feeling, sensory and motor impulses. The regulation of these lies within every one of us who wants to tune his motor, rather than depend on a pill as a weak substitute for personal effort and understanding applied to ourself. Our mind always wants to escape, rather than apply itself to the problem and solve it by continued concentrated effort.

Electromagnetic Light Waves and Their Chemical Effect Upon Cells

Health is the neutral position in life by which the cellular activity of the body is in a neutral polarity state called balance. In this state the energies of the body are in tune and in communication with all life in the cosmos and exchange freely in etheric and airy essences, and elements so vital to health, through a balanced flow of electromagnetic light waves, like rivers from a universal ocean of supply. Then life flows unconscious of itself in an exuberant expression as in childhood. There is no interference from positive or negative energy blocks, because the currents flow in harmony like the alternating electric currents in light and power production, without shorts or ground leakage.

This is the energy that flows from the brain like a central light wave, the Thousand Petalled Lotus,* of the primal electromagnetic energy radiating from the top of the head, at the fontanels (in childhood), downward and outward like the lotus of life. This tree of life sustains the body through the brain, the spinal cord, and the entire nervous system.

---

*Thousand Petalled Lotus: According to the Hindu tradition, this vision appears to religious devotees who, through meditation, are able to concentrate and focus all their attention at the Third Eye at the center of the forehead.

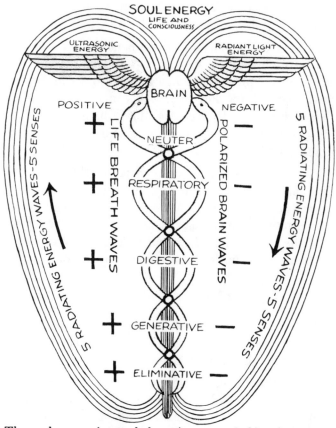

The caduceus pictured above* was carried by the messenger of the God of life, called Hermes by the Greeks and Egyptians and Mercury by the Romans, always pictured with wings on his feet. The caduceus was the symbol of healing for the physicians of old, who understood some of this mystery of life and applied it in their limited way. A globe with two wings symbolizes the two hemispheres of the brain, with a central staff or trunk of this tree of life, which is the spinal cord. The two life-breaths wind down this tree of life as two serpents of mind and emotional impulses, or energy fields expressed in their stepped-down energy as the two life-breaths,

---

*This illustration is from Dr. Stone's book *Polarity Therapy*. Various charts and illustrations of this principle are also found in his book *The Wireless Anatomy of Man* (e.g., chart 12 on "the tree of life").

positive and negative, flowing through the right and left nostrils, called Pingala (or Yang) and Ida (or Yin).*

This is also the story of Prometheus Bound who brought this flame of life down to mankind and suffered for it. It is the story of all humanity when understood, and the electromagnetic light waves and their fields in the cells tell us how this occurs in us, with every rhythmic breath, thought, and feeling or impulse. It is the story of our life told simply; it is the subject of health and life.

Positive and negative electromagnetic light waves connect our life and energy principle with the whole cosmic supply in space, as the primary respiration, while our breathing in and out connects us with the earth's atmosphere and exchange of gases of the carbon dioxide in our lungs for oxygen and nitrogen combination. This is the secondary respiration.

Cellular Effects

Cells are affected two ways by the energy of electromagnetic light waves. When they become imbalanced in their charge, they are the primary cause of disease.

1. A concentration of electromagnetic light wave energy with an increase of hydrogen ions deposited in the cell makes the cell over-acid in its chemistry and produces acute symptoms of redness, heat, swelling and inflammation. These symptoms are an excess of positive charge and the action of the fire principle,† which produces acute diseases, which are mostly self-limiting and corrective in Nature's effort to restore life, where obstruction was present. Fevers have a remedial effect when understood and handled correctly and wisely.

---

*Pingala (or Yang) and Ida (or Yin): This concept of the two life-breaths weaving as currents of energy down the spine is central to both Indian and Chinese spiritual and healing traditions.

† Fire principle: The principle of heat and expansion in all living things.

2. *A deconcentration* of electromagnetic light waves in the fields of the cells with an increase of hydroxyl ions makes the cells excessively alkaline, cold, constricted and dehydrated. This is the basis for all chronic diseases and limitation of motion. Here the water element* is functioning in excess, as the primary polarity factor in the energy fields' imbalance, as an excess negative charge with its constrictive over-alkalinity, limiting function and motion, and its crippling effect like in arthritis, rheumatism, etc.

Depressed and *repressed* mental-emotional states have an effect on the electromagnetic waves and their charge and cellular polarity. These fields can be balanced when the patient is co-operative and willing to work with it as change in diet, habits, hot and cold water therapy, sunbaths, grounding the body, etc. But primarily it is the new inspiration of hope and a positive attitude that makes the vital change in the mental, emotional ion attraction and polarity fields of the electromagnetic light wave charges. It is here where the humorous element comes in to arouse the patient by making him good and mad, so he or she will show you what they can do. The stories of the effectiveness of this suggestive therapy are legion and most practical when used with discretion. The inspiration given by new ideas, new hopes, a new doctor, a new cure all have the same basic impact in the energy field on a stagnant, negatively-charged mind and emotion with its deteriorating chemistry. We are either self-motivated or we must be pushed. This finer chemistry, connected with our emotions and thinking, has not been given much attention and yet is one of the greatest factors in our life and health-building process. "As a man thinketh, so is he." Every cell responds to the pattern-energy impulse. The process of breathing sustains our life in the earth's atmosphere. We depend on every breath to sustain us in that moment of life on earth. If

---

*Water element: The principle of fluidity and cooling in nature.

that process stops, we have had it. The same can be said for our thinking and emotional impulses which proceed from within us through the cerebrospinal fluid conduction and can be tuned to higher life ideals which overcome many limitations and effects.

Tuning in with the Infinite is a practical idea, if applied and understood. Man is not as helpless as he feels and thinks he is, if he could only tune in on his inner energies and deeper hidden resources of life itself. Life is the Unit Cause; effects are endless and we lose ourselves in them; we look to effects for our help and remedies, rather than to life itself and to the cosmic whole of the manifesting energy called Nature.

Our mental and emotional energies become chemistry by the attraction of space particles or ions, through our electromagnetic light waves and fields. This fact will awaken us with a shock to the truth that our condition proceeds from life and its conditioning within ourselves through mental and emotional impulses. We can rebuild and mold our body daily psychologically as well as physiologically. Enervation through physical exhaustion or excesses are real factors of disease and often develop from a mental background.

First things first even in health-building: understanding and purpose are the blueprints of our life; the body is our garden and house which we must care for if we want to live in it. So we select the right food (fuel) which we can easily digest and which has all the finer natural elements in its uncooked state for replacing worn-out elements and tissues. The stomach is our carburetor which must not be flooded. The right combination of foods helps to blend the chemistry in the process of digestion. The wrong combinations or excess food cause fermentation and gas. The symptom of backfiring is not only the trouble of engines alone. Carbon dioxide is a natural by-product of combustion. It keeps the intestines and colon inflated so they won't stick together or kink and form obstructions. There is a natural compensatory arrangement between the CO_2 in the bowels and in the blood stream.

Often acute high blood pressure symptoms are due to gas in the circulation and are not serious at all, as it can be released quickly. Most headaches are due to gas in the bloodstream. Oxydation is caused by the moisture effect in the process of combustion. Good digestion produces good oxydation and elimination. It is important to know how these vital effects all hang together on the one process—digestion, which is the fire element in action in the body. From all this we can see the vital importance of wise and careful eating for health to extend our span of life and health. Life is a gift from the Beloved Creator. Like wealth, we can waste it, spend it fast, or use it wisely and conservatively and live longer. We can dig our grave prematurely by reckless habits of wasting the energies of life, and with the fork and knife as bad eating habits.

Our every action is our karma, which decides our life here. We are either a wise steward or an inefficient manager. How often do we not have proof of this, when we see a handicapped person or a sickly one do better and live longer than a robust healthy-looking one? To give just one example, Frank Gotch, the world's outstanding wrestler, died at the age of 42. On the other hand the great scientist Tyndal, who was so weak physically that he could not even carry his big dictionary from one place to another in the room, lived to a ripe old age. And among handicapped persons, we need only mention Helen Keller to prove what effort and will can accomplish. With these facts and proof, no one can glory in his ill health or in his appendix operation. Clear thinkers try to find the causes, while the average look for escapes from effects.

This puts the whole picture into a different light as to causes, which lie in ourselves, rather than in some germ. Humanity must grow up sometime and be responsible for its action in war or peace. Only when we understand ourselves can we get along with ourselves and value this precious gift of life, given for the sole purpose of freeing our Soul and consciousness from the snares of the mind and senses, which are the real cause of our suffering and ill health. The outer evidences are but the symptoms of the inner conflicts of energies and inharmony. The old hermetic law declared this Truth:

> *As above so below.*
> *As within so without.*

All things except the wind cast their shadow. No one can compel us to think or to live the truth we know. "A man convinced against his will is of the same opinion still." If we do not understand ourselves and our problem of ill health, then who can solve it for us, if we don't change the cause of it in ourselves? Surely, we can go to doctors and take medicines for a long time without touching the inner causes of the energy fields and our habits and diet.

When will we grow up and really think? And make a supreme effort to return to the Father's House, whence our consciousness descended? True health is the harmony of life within us and is happiness and well-being. Merely having no pain is not always a happy condition of the mind and of life. We are entitled to more and if we look for it, we will find it. These truths are for the few and not for the multitude. But if a person suffers, he must think and find an answer; and this does not always lie waiting for us in the chemist's shop. Life proves it.

Now for some further practical help in illness and disease. The logical thing to do first would be to stop eating like the animals do. Then rest and think and wash out the debris of the system from above and below. The basic goal is to get the energies to flow; as the gross substance and gases move on, there will be relief. Nature is not in a hurry, neither can we be. We conserve energy when we stop eating. It takes a lot of energy to digest food and distribute it and get rid of it again. We should employ Nature's energies to balance themselves by first taking off the load and stress. A motor will idle nicely when it has no load to pull. Use Nature to help you. It does all the healing anyway, so why make it always react to medicines and injections, increasing the load it has to bear? Why not give Nature the chance to heal in the first place?

The electromagnetic fields will balance themselves as a rule, if given a chance Nature's way. Quieting the emotions by faith, hope, and love is most helpful. Water cleanses and rest restores weakened magnetic fields, and makes us think; which alone can remove many a kink. But everybody thinks, we must do something to stop the symptoms instead of giving Nature a chance to clean house. Can an outsider know more than Nature within of the obstacles and energy blocks which confront it? If we could but be really still and get in touch with this inner life, the answer would readily appear as in any good computer when the right question is put in. We have the best built-in computer on earth and we do not know it or use it.

When the body is in a state of perfect rest, then the computer life-principle within works with its own problem and acts, if it is not interfered with or burdened with food. To get good advice is excellent but to act on it and understand the problem is better. When no answer is found, then these things which I have written here apply. We must dig deep and find the life energy and engage its attention and assist Nature's process of elimination, oxidation, circulation, liver function, bowel and kidney action, etc. Nature is grand, if we but understand.

4

The New Age & Polarity Therapy

"Ability and skill are developed by effort and experience, not by talk. . . . We get so much education nowadays that we don't know what's real anymore!"

We are in the sign of Aquarius, the water bearer, the carrier of the water of space energy and its truth. It is a new age of technology with rapid changes and progress. Mankind has seen the vision of space as a larger horizon of life in usefulness, with better understanding dawning on the minds of humanity.

The useless cruelty of man and the bitter lessons of suffering and loss of life, property, and mounting costs into future generations have taken the edge off nationality fixations and war. Technocracy is intriguing to the minds of the younger generation, even in totalitarian countries.

The frantic research in atomic science and its progress have ushered in a new age of the ever-becoming usefulness of things through a better knowledge of the energy factors in matter and in life. Beautiful doodles of lines of force and the mathematics of proportion confront us in all research. The science of energy with its electronic and atomic research is the key to this new age.

Research

For more than 45 years, I have been making research into energy fields in their relation to the healing art. I started with the life principle in the center and worked outward in its application. I studied most of the ancient concepts of life and their approach to the life in man as an energy radiation principle in Nature in relation to the unit of life in man. It was called odic fluid, mesmerism, animal magnetism, and many other names. Man's constitution in the finer energy fields of mind, emotions, electromagnetic light waves, radiations and their effect on the chemistry in the cell as polarity energy of attraction and repulsion is the reality behind these names.

All cells are bipolar or they could not act and function. The law of polarity—of positive, negative and neuter energy—rules all matter as the principle of the three gunas from the mind downward. Attraction and repulsion is the manifestation of life, as sex-polarity of male and female through all creation of vegetation, animals and humans. Even metals have their positive and negative polarity, values like the gold and silver which attract the sun and moon energies and are fine conductors for electronic constructions. Much silver is being used for it now.

In this research, I have stumbled onto a science which blends the old concept of energies in the constitution of man and have linked it with the scientific research in space as the magnetosphere and electromagnetic lines of force in man's constitution. In my books and courses for doctors, I had drawings made which outline this in detail in relationship to the anatomy and physiology of the body. This relationship is the art of Polarity Therapy, based on the primary mind pattern energy in the brain which is duplicated in every oval of the body* as the five bases for sensory perception and motor function by which we live and act. Near as it is to us, it is nevertheless a lost art, once called the Spagyric Art by the great medieval Doctor Paracelsus von Hoenheim. He was taught its secrets in Arabia and in other parts of the then-travelled world, even among shepherds and gypsies who lived near the

---

*Oval of the body: Dr. Stone refers here to the five ovals of the torso: the head, the neck, the chest, the abdomen and the pelvis.

grass roots of life with some strange traditions and secrets from the past. It became a lost art again after the great doctor passed on in Salzburg, Austria, on September 24, 1541.

His great contribution was the use of the electromagnetic energy waves to human chemistry. His research and knowledge in chemistry gave a great boost to that science, but the real secret of the electromagnetic energy connection with chemistry was lost to the world. Only chemistry in its grosser form survived and the world benefited by it.

*Polarity Therapy** is the name I gave to this art of correspondences of body spaces and functions, through attraction and repulsion of electromagnetic energy waves as the roots of the five senses—sensory and motor—functioning in the body. Linking it with the cerebrospinal fluid radiation and circulation brought it into the realm of physiology and through the brain, the spinal cord and nerves and its meningeal coverings made it a tangible asset in research and in practice of the Healing Art. Polarity Therapy provides a definite location for the electromagnetic fields and their directive life-giving energy in man, which can be used as a definite art in therapeutics.

To help others by means of these new principles of polarity, I have travelled around the world three times and treated many patients, mostly in India as I stayed there longest for the study of depth perception in life called Spirituality by the Masters. In Dera Baba Jaimal Singh Colony near Beas, district of Amritsar in the Punjab, I held large free clinics to help the helpless and hopeless cases. As a result, I am known from Bombay to Calcutta and wherever I go, patients are waiting for me as their last hope, and I only take cases that have failed to respond to all other methods of treatments. This I consider a fair test of Polarity Therapy as I have not merely followed precedents and the regular accepted routine of any one system, even in the manipulative arts of Osteopathy, Chiropractic, Naprapathy or any mechanotherapy.

---

*Many of the specifics about Polarity Therapy mentioned in this chapter can only be clearly understood by studying Dr. Stone's advanced books on the subject and by learning the procedures from an experienced Polarity Therapy teacher.

Body Polarity Applied

The human body is bipolar like the cell. This applies to the anatomy and the physiological function as well. The anatomy forms the fields of location and relationships, while the physiology follows the cerebrospinal fluid radiations in their functions as electromagnetic waves, and can be applied as therapy with the hands as polarity of positive and negative poles. In studying this I found the key to craniopathy, which moves the cranial bones by application of the skill of the hands to the head.

The science of Polarity Therapy can be proved by therapy applications of electromagnetic energy waves through the right and left hands to opposite parts of any area in its three dimensions of space: anterior and posterior, superior and inferior, and from side to side. Not only does the brain energy in the cranium affect the body and move cranial bones, it also sets the brain and the spinal cord into rhythmic vibrating waves, which can be felt by sensitive patients; but conversely, body areas set the brain in motion and can be felt by patients. It has been proven definitely on cases of serious eye trouble where even cortisone therapy in hospitals could not relieve and save the eye function. I speak of eye cases, because definite checks have been made by the optometrist on his modern machines of testing the eyes and using pictures for eye exercise through muscle training.

Toxicity

Only by working with sick patients can one see how toxic they are and how this toxin has settled more heavily on some area where the pain is, where the cerebrospinal fluid is obstructed by the toxic material and its resistance as a nonconductor of energy currents. It is here that Polarity Therapy as a principle can be applied to great advantage to help the patient, especially when he is too sick or too much in pain for any manipulative type of therapy. Only after the cerebro-spinal fluid current is established is there a beneficial reaction to any application of therapy.

It is this energy current which does the healing and reacts to therapy. No adjustments can be given with a good reaction where the cerebrospinal fluid is not active. This has puzzled chiropractors for a long time—why the same adjustments have such a different reaction at different times even on the same patient.

If we have the key to unlock the core,
We find Nature standing at the door!

It is here that polarizing the three nervous systems is of the greatest benefit for the patient.

1. Balance the sensory parasympathetic 10th cranial nerve currents to release tension and spasm.

2. Release the 11th cranial nerve current.

3. Release the hypersensitive magnetic fields where spinal anemia keeps them from functioning.

This is found at the tip of the spinous processes where there is great hypersensitiveness with the vasodilators over-active on the surface, and anemia in the center. Cold quick applications or alcohol applied here will be very effective. The left hand over it, and the right hand opposite to it is good therapy. Polarity Therapy affects the movement of the cerebro-spinal fluid directly. Manipulation and hot and cold affect the circulation through dilation and constriction of the vaso-motor system. Drugs can also act as a stimulant or as a depress-ing agent, where there is enough current for a reaction.

The key to the cell and to the body is through the cerebro-spinal fluid energy currents. Polarity currents applied are most direct, gentle and very effective. They can start a flow where it has been interrupted. A yawn, a deep sigh, a twitch or gentle perspiration verifies the balance of relaxation estab-lished. Then, any indicated adjustment will give good results.

Eyes can be strengthened by head polarization, and tension and pain relieved by polarizing the 4th toe or by holding both toes on top of the feet and the arch interspaces for five minutes.

5

Health-Building Diet

"We want to dominate and tell God what to do—after misusing what He gave us. . . . I used to run the universe, and then I got out of it. Now it runs better!"

Food and drink are the fuel for our bodily functions. Air and warmth are the combustion factors of our motor. There are four stages of this process: 1. Digestion, 2. Assimilation, 3. Elimination, and 4. Oxidation. When any one of these processes is incomplete, the body suffers. Therefore, it is essential for us to take only the foods and drinks which can be digested fully in the stomach, chemicalized by the liver, absorbed by the intestines, and eliminated by the colon. Then only will the oxidation be completed through the skin and the lungs in a normal way.

The stomach is the digestive center on the left side of the body, and the liver is the big chemical organ on the right side. When these two function normally, then the digestive process in its lysis (or breaking down of the food into its component elements and the subsequent chemical reassembling of elements and their change into bodily materials) will be completed in harmony of function.

But when there is a constant overload and too rich a fuel (too much and too rich a food), then these two polarity functions break down and the whole economy of the body suffers and goes wrong. So the first step in retracing is to clear these two functions and to give the body a chance to right itself in its own chemistry without drugs.

In choosing a diet, we must think of the real requirements of the body and find the natural foods which contain all the

36

enzymes, the vitamins and minerals which the body needs. Merely satisfying the appetite and old habits or customs is not enough when we want to get well and have started out on a Health-Building Program. It is like building a house; we must have good material. And people who need this most cannot afford to buy expensive enzymes to aid digestion, nor the vitamins needed daily for the tissues and nerves as well as the minerals to replace those lost by wear and tear and through elimination and oxidation. So they will have to choose natural fruits, grains, greens and vegetables and nuts which contain all these elements in their sealed-in compartments, waiting to be used.

Any good fresh fruit or uncooked greens constitute nature's eliminative diet. This can be improved by using almond oil, olive oil, sesame oil, or sunflower seed oil, etc., with garlic and lime juice added as a salad dressing. Garlic in oil is a valuable addition. It can be peeled and put right into the cruet with the oil to give it flavor and additional value without being detected on the breath. The garlic loses its flavor in the oil in about one week and should be exchanged for fresh garlic before it turns color, to keep the oil potentized with the garlic essence. The lemon or lime is always used fresh squeezed as needed. It is added to the oil just before using it, as the citrus juice rapidly loses its value once it is extracted.

Juices
Never let fresh fruit juices stand after they are squeezed out because they oxidize and lose value every minute they are exposed to the air. The moment the hermetic seal of the fruit or vegetable is broken, it must be used, if you want to get the full value of its fine trace elements, enzymes and some of the vitamins which oxidize readily. All fruit juices or cut fruits will deteriorate when exposed to the air. They change in chemical value also, and have a tendency to turn sour. Do not cut the fruits until you are ready to use them at once, or mix them with oil for the salad. All fresh uncooked greens provide the needed chlorophyll.

Enzymes, Vitamins and Minerals

To obtain these for home use from your ordinary grains is a simple matter that takes just a little work and extra care in preparation. Sprout your grains or legumes: the beans, peas, lentils, garbanzos, foenugreek seeds, alfalfa seeds, millet, wheat, oats, barley, rye, buckwheat, corn or sprouts of any other edible grains or seeds, except the tomato or the potato which are not edible as sprouts.

You not only save on quantity if you sprout grains and seeds and then chew them raw. You also have all the life elements and protein you need without cooking them or overloading your stomach or being constantly hungry after eating even a big meal of cooked food. The body needs these fine live ingredients which are lost in cooking, and their need is felt by the sensory mechanism as an unsatisfied wanting of something more. And quantities of cooked food only overload the stomach and ferment, causing bloating and wind.

For Children and Grown-Ups

Getting the latent life-elements plus the protein in the food, included in the live sprouts and tender greens, is very important for health. In sprouting you have set Nature's entire chain reaction of reproduction to work for you, and you get the full benefit when you eat the sprouts or tender greens. Little is needed for the best results. You are dealing with life's power of reproduction. And for children that are undernourished or always hungry and pale, what could you give them at any time without the trouble of cooking or much cost than some of these sprouted grains or seeds with honey over it, or a little oil with garlic and honey. It is very tasty when chewed and most satisfying as a meal or in between. These sprouts will keep for several days in a refrigerator or cool place and are always ready for use. Simply put them in a glass jar with a lid on and your reserve is ready.

A *vitality drink* can be made from the sprouts, young wheat grass or other edible greens by liquidizing a cupful of alfalfa or foenugreek sprouts, etc., and combining it with some pineapple juice or other fruit juice, sweetened with honey to taste. It is a great pick-up for new energy. There would be less drunkenness in the world if the body's real needs were supplied with such an invigorating drink when there was a craving for alcohol or a stimulant.

Serving Combinations for Guests

Grind together equal parts of any sprout, say wheat with almonds or cashew nuts, and seeded raisins. Form it into rolls or sticks and roll in fresh grated coconut and honey. Salads can be made very quickly in the absence of other greens with about one pint of foenugreek, alfalfa or millet sprouts with diced avocadoes, cucumbers, tomatoes, etc. Toss and serve with sesame seed oil with garlic in it and season with fresh lime juice and honey as a dressing when it is served.

Other combinations offer endless possibilities, such as finely chopped soy or mung bean sprouts with fresh potato patties, sour cream dressing or yogurt or curd besides. Season sprout dishes with herbs, such as sweet basil, or any herb seasoning you like. It is best not to cook the sprouts, as you lose the enzymes of life and vitamins. Sprouts can be added to any cooked vegetables or other food when served, to assure the supply of the elements missing in cooked food alone. New combinations are a discovery for everyone.

Choice of Sprouts

Foenugreek or alfalfa seeds are chosen for their eliminative quality, high mineral content and ease in handling. They are excellent for rheumatics and ill persons. In South Africa, ostrich raisers observed stronger young ones and better plumage if they are fed on young alfalfa grass. Arabs observed the same results for their horses. It made them more lithe and faster, and it did the same for men. Because of this, they called it al-fal-fa—father of all foods. The main reason for this is that it sends its little rootlets so deep into the earth that some were found as far as 60 feet down at times, to gather minerals and earthy essences of rare value.

Alfalfa contains vitamin B complex, B8, vitamin K, the blood-clotting vitamin; also potassium, phosphorus, and calcium, which are essential minerals needed for tissue building, brain function and bone, teeth and blood building.

All sprouting is done best in the dark, in a warm place and by steady moisture. The seeds must be washed three or four times a day to free them of slime. They must never be allowed to get dry. And they must not stand in water while sprouting or they will sour. Perfect drainage is essential at all times while sprouting any seeds.

Sprouting Seeds for Food

First, soak the seeds to be sprouted for 12 hours—overnight. Then place them about two or three thick, one-eighth of an inch or so, on the bottom of a container with fine holes in it for good drainage. A plastic screen is ideal for this purpose. A wooden bowl or a strainer, or a fine wire mesh screen is all that is needed, with a cloth on the bottom and top, or a clay tray with a hole in it will do. If the holes are too large, a layer of cloth is necessary to keep the seeds and moisture in. They are then covered with a wet cloth, doubled, to hold steady moisture. Keep in the dark and warm. Wash the seeds three times a day with a pressure spray hose, if you have it, to get the slime off; otherwise, dump the seeds into a strainer and wash the bottom and top cloth well and wash the seeds in the strainer with cool running water and put them back on the cloth in the tray.

A tray or strainer with fine holes saves all that work when washing them, because it needs no cloth below; but only a double or triple thickness on the top to keep the seeds moist. In 72 hours, you will have fine sprouts, ready for use or storage in your refrigerator or in a cool place when put into a jar. They will keep for several days, if kept cool.

Sprouting Wheat Grass
for Chlorophyll and Greens Only

Soak the seeds first—overnight—12 hours, then sow them. For this you use mother earth, a little space of a few square feet in the garden in good soil. Have several sections so you can change off, planting one while harvesting the other. You can have boxes of flower pots with earth in them for this purpose all the year around. It will grow without sunshine, if this is not available. Four to six inches of good earth is sufficient. Use a few earthworms in the box also and put any pressed-out greens, when making juice of it only, back and mix with the earth. It acts like a compost to the soil. Leaf mold soil from under the trees is the best earth for this.

Keep the earth moist; you can harvest the greens in seven days. It can be cut three times and then replanted. The grass can be from four to seven inches tall when cut; the young sprouts are most tender. They can be chewed like gum and the benefit absorbed, and the residue, if there is any, can be spit out. This green can be combined with anything to enrich the meal, but is best by itself when chewed very carefully or chopped up fine into salads, or in drinks mixed with pineapple or fruit juices. It can be added to soup when served and to other foods as a finely chopped green dressing. It contains the much-needed finer elements and chlorophyll so vital to life.

Foods have a polarity as acid and alkaline, by which they act and react on each other during the process of digestion and can cause fermentation and souring in the stomach. Therefore, acid foods, such as citrus fruits, and sour foods containing vinegar, should not be combined with starches, like bread, cake, cereals or grains of any kind, nor with potatoes or rice. Orange juice and cereals dry or cooked are a bad combination unless the citrus juice is taken on an empty stomach one-half hour before the breakfast. Sweet fruits and juices, such as figs, dates, raisins, prunes and prune juice, combine well with cereals.

Starchy food should be chewed well so that the saliva mixes with it and prepares it for further digestion in the intestines by mixing it with the enzyme of ptyalin in the saliva, which acts upon the starches. That is why all the grass and grain-eating animals spend so much time in chewing their food. They grind it up thoroughly and mix it with saliva, to stay well; and they do, if the food is suitable and provides all the elements needed for life's process. But man hasn't time for that, so he spends months in hospitals to try to patch up what a disregard for Nature's law of life brought on.

Protein foods and acids are agreeable and a good combination because they both take acid media for their digestion and thus will not cause fermentation by souring through an alkaline-acid reaction between them in digesting. Protein foods and starchy food are a bad combination, such as meat or eggs with bread, since the proteins require the acid in the stomach for their digestion. The starches are absorbent like a sponge and take up that liquid and cannot use it, since they are digested by the saliva in the mouth and, in the small intestines, by the amylopsin and diastase enzymes. Starches eaten with proteins, then, delay the digestion and cause fermentation.

Milk is a baby food. It should not be taken with other proteins at any meal. Two types of proteins are excessive and delay the digestion. The old Jewish law would never allow milk on the table with their big meal of the day. Milk is best combined with starches—potatoes, cereals, bread—and sweet fruits. Sour milk and yogurt are better for adults than sweet milk, as they are partly cheese already. *Vegetables* are best combined with all *proteins* either as a cooked dish or as a *raw* salad. That is an ideal combination for all big meals.

Liquids—Persons with poor digestion should not take liquids with meals, as they dilute the digestive juices and thus delay the digestion, causing bloating and headaches. For the same reason, cold drinks should not be taken with meals. They also chill the stomach below the normal point of 105 degrees Fahrenheit at which digestion takes place and thus delay the digestive process in two ways: by dilution and by temperature lowering delaying the chemical process.

Most headaches after meals are due to one or more of these improper combinations of foods. Gases in the blood are the causes of most headaches; gas is absorbed by the bloodstream from the fermentations in the process of digestion and from food particles taken into the circulation when in a state of fermentation and incomplete digestion. These are the trouble makers which can go on for years and lead to all kinds of pain symptoms and disease, until the cause is discovered and the diet corrected. That is why fasting for a few days on water and papaya, or fruit juices helps to clear the bloodstream of these foreign objects and catch up on its delayed digestive process. Fasting also aids elimination of the accumulated material, the wastes in the circulation and in the tissue cells where it is packed away and stored until a health crisis, when it will be activated and cause acute symptoms.

The "why" is forgotten and the process is considered as a devastating disease when all one needs is no food and cold packs to keep the skin active to oxidize the waste and to control the fever which is the overactive digestive process. When the fire of digestion becomes overactive, it means that there is rubbish somewhere which needs burning up, oxidizing and neutralizing. But it is not normally recognized in this capacity as a healing factor in the body's economy. We want to direct Nature's economy from the outside and we interfere with life's fire element in its course of action, like stopping someone from burning up their own rubbish.

We readily agree that clothes need washing to be clean but we do not give that privilege to the tissues in the body, and so we create many varieties of diseases by suppression of Nature's natural process of burning its rubbish. No chronic disease can be cured without an acute effort by our inner intelligence and a fever to raise the tissues into life again by a better and stronger circulation and inner warmth, thus linking it back to the active life process within.

"Man rushes in where angels fear to tread," but the learned intellect does not understand life and its process as a unit action and reaction. Intellect divides and aims to rule in parts. There is no end of diseases, because of the emphasis on detail of parts and description, like the leaves on a single tree. Life is one, and its process is one. Otherwise, the many parts would never make up a whole again as a unit of life. All this hangs together as one of the Polarity functions of the fire element. If I were to say it was the god Shiva in action, many in India would agree with me and would not try to suppress him or his ways of ruling life; but a little learning is a dangerous thing.

Many good farmers feed their animals much more carefully and better than they do their families. Animals cost money and they understand them much better than they do themselves, their wives, or their children's real need of wholesome natural food with life elements in it.

Helpful Suggestions to Regain Health and Overcome Diabetes

The liver is the largest organ in the body and is the key to its chemical function. That is why the liver should be considered in the selection of our diet and should be assisted when its function is impeded or subnormal.

Excessive use of sugar is hard on the liver, as it must convert all this into glycogen and then store it for use, by means of its chemical function. The same can be said about excessive intake of starches. The saliva and the pancreatic juice convert starches into maltose and then into dextrose. Now, supposing the starchy food is not thoroughly masticated but is gulped down or washed down with liquids, what becomes of this neglected process, when the liver has to handle the food, improperly prepared for the next chemical change? Is it any wonder that diabetes sets in because a person tries to live on cooked food alone and much starchy food which is not thoroughly masticated nor properly insalivated because the food is mixed with liquids and seemingly needs no chewing?

What else can nature do when one complete process like insalivation does not support the other processes of natural function? Also, when the diet is excessively rich in cooked, starchy foods and sweets, and contains no green sprouts, no salads and little fruit, from where will nature get her needed materials? And when the disease sets in, we test for the symptoms and treat the effect successfully for a lifetime, but forget the cause completely and think we are serving Nature and humanity!

Fats: No fried food should be eaten because that clogs the liver and makes heavy demands on its functioning. The liver must break up the fat-soaked particles which are amalgamated by a temperature of from 200 to 450 degrees F. and try to separate the fats from the food with a normal liver temperature of 107 degrees F. Dizziness, headaches and spots before the eyes are a few mild symptoms of this malfunction.

Some fats are used for cooking repeatedly until they are used up, and more is added, like the hot fats doughnuts and French fries are cooked in. Those are overheated, dead fats and we eat them cooked into foods like doughnuts, French fried potatoes, roasted nuts, etc. Butter, when heated over a certain degree, breaks down into oleic and stearic acid. It cannot stand the high heat that other animal fats or oils can tolerate. Butterfat is not ideal for cooking for that reason. Uncooked, it has good food value; cooked, it is the worst fat for the liver to handle because of its chemical break-down. Many people have suffered because of this without even knowing it, as it is a common daily practice. Even cancer has been traced to the frequent use of overheated fats like lard and cottonseed oil. And we think diseases run in families when they all eat the same! Why not? The cause is obvious and does not need the help of germs.

Oils: Cold-pressed almond oil has very good value for the liver and bowels. Also cold-pressed olive oil, sesame oil, sunflower seed oil, safflower oil and corn oil. Without heating, the oil is an antidote for the liver which is clogged from overheated oil products and with fresh lime or lemon juice, three times as much as the oil, a fine liver flush is made. So I call it the "liver-flush" and use it in the morning before or instead of tea.

6

Diet & Health: A Daily Diet to Regain Health*

"We know so much about disease, but nothing about health! Don't treat disease; treat the individual. Find out where the energy is blocked!"

The first thing in the morning, instead of bed tea, I recommend a "liver-flush" to bring it back to its normal function.

1. *Liver-flush:* From one to three tablespoonfuls of pure, cold pressed almond or olive oil mixed with thrice the amount of fresh lime or lemon juice—stir and drink it. Then take two cupfuls of *hot* water with the juice of one-half or a whole lime or lemon to each cupful.

   Alternative: One glassful (8 ounces) *fresh* orange, grapefruit, pomegranate or pineapple juice may be taken with the oil and followed by the two cupfuls of *hot* lemon water.

   Constipation is also relieved by either of the above practices.

2. *Breakfast:* For a quick cleansing, diet should consist of only fresh fruits, such as papaya with lemon on it, apples, pears, guavas, oranges, pomegranates, or melons, apricots,

---

*The dietary principles in this chapter may be applied generally for most conditions. See Chapter 14 for a specific outline of a more rigorous "Purifying Diet."

grapes, or raisins. A few almonds can be added and chewed well.

Breakfast of a more substantial nature for workers: one hour or more *after* the liver-flush, or when the almond oil is no longer needed, then *one* hour or more *after* taking the hot lime or lemon water and honey, take half a cup of freshly pressed out ginger juice combined with a cup of hot water in which raisins, dates or figs were soaked all night. Put the soaked fruit in the porridge. Then have a liberal helping of porridge made of three-fourths millet and one-fourth foenugreek seeds well cooked and with some raisins in it. A banana, some honey or guava jam, not too sweet, or any naturally sweet fruit may be taken with the porridge—BUT NEVER a citrus fruit. Also have one or two dozen peeled almonds and masticate them well. This makes a very substantial breakfast. Chew it well.

3. *Beverages:* Under no circumstances should one ever partake of alcoholic drinks. Not only does alcohol give one a false sense of well-being, followed by mental depression, but it also dulls the brain and pickles the food in the stomach, causing indigestion. Alcohol is also hard on the liver and kidneys.

    Take hot water with lime or lemon and honey in it to sweeten to taste and to act as a cleanser for the blood-stream. Soak raisins, figs, dates and almonds, drink the water and use the fruits.

    For a daily beverage, instead of coffee or regular tea, make a tea from ginger root, foenugreek seeds and peppermint; sweeten with honey and flavour with lemon or lime juice.

    A glass of *fresh* orange or grapefruit juice in between meals is very beneficial. It contains vitamin C in abundance if taken immediately after extracting the juice. It should not be allowed to stand, as the longer it is exposed, the more it loses of its value. The natural fruit sugar is levulose and is easily digested and assimilated.

4. *Between Meals:* While on the cleansing diet (number 1 & 2), if hungry, take hot water with lemon and honey in it instead of coffee or tea and sugar or other snacks. Sugar is usually used in excess in coffee, tea and the daily diet. This is bad for the liver and pancreas, and leads to diabetes. Use honey instead of sugar wherever possible. You need very little sweets and no sugar.

   Any fresh fruit may be taken between meals, whenever one is hungry.

5. *Noon Meal:* Steamed, boiled or baked vegetables and beans. Sprout them first, then use them. They have the most value when chewed without cooking them (beans, peas, lentils, lima beans, chick peas all belong to this group).

   Legumes are rich in protein and are far superior to meat and eggs, as they do not contain the harmful by-products. CHEESE is also rich in protein and can be used with any meal, whether with vegetables or fruit, but it should not be cooked or baked, as it loses value and is hard to digest after it has been subjected to too much heat. Cheese, fruits and vegetables which have not been cooked, pasteurized or subjected to too high a temperature (not over 118 degrees F.) contain enzymes, which are essential for digestion. Hence, salads of fresh fruits or fresh vegetables and fresh sprouts from the legumes, the grains and foenugreek are highly recommended and preferable to cooked foods. You get more enzymes and vitamins that way.

6. *Evening Meal:* Should be light and not too late. Heavy and late meals are bad for health, add to weight and sluggishness, and are responsible for inefficiency the next day.

   Any fresh fruit or combination of fresh fruits and warm milk make a choice evening meal for one who is exhausted, ill, nervous or suffers from digestive trouble and sleeplessness.

For a more substantial evening meal, rolled oats (Quaker oats, etc.) or wheat porridge and fresh sweet fruit or raisins, figs, dates or prunes, and honey are recommended, the same as for breakfast, except that the almonds may be omitted at night.

Caution: Do not eat anything fried nor cooked in fat of any kind, as that makes the food too rich and indigestible, causing fermentation. Much rheumatism is due to fermentation in the system as a result of this practice.

Instead: Add some butter, or better still, some sesame oil, olive oil, almond oil or any good vegetable oil with lemon to taste, to the food as it is served. Preferably, allow each one to add this to his own portion of food, so that the amount may be according to the individual's taste and needs.

Caution: Never drink cold water, iced tea, etc., after the meals; it slows down the process of digestion. The stomach works at 105 degrees F.

Instead: One may take fresh ginger juice with the meal, sufficient to suit the taste and aid digestion. For a hot drink, if one is desired with the meal, use the tea made of ginger, foenugreek and peppermint, sweetened with honey.

Some good whole-wheat bread or toast may be taken sparingly. Bake your own whole-wheat or rye barley bread. But note that wheat, corn, millet, etc. are best cooked as porridge and more easily digested that way. It is soaked thoroughly and cooked longer.

Note: Only sweet fruits combine with cereals. Never combine acids and starches; that is, citrus fruit or juices (oranges, grapefruit, lemons, limes) should *never* be taken *with* the starches nor after a meal consisting of any starchy food (potatoes, rice and all cereals, bread), because it sours the food and causes fermentation, which is the background of many a case of arthritis and rheumatism.

Man's body, emotions and mind are a part of Nature and need constantly to be in tune with Nature to attract their supply for sustenance, breath, warmth and moisture for growth and life. Food and liquids supply the earthy elements of replacement for the structure. Air and warmth of sunshine supply the energy elements of motion and function.

When these energy currents flow freely without interruption there is a state of balance by being in tune with Nature, which is freedom of motion and function, called health. But any interference in this natural flow of energy manifests as a multitude of pains and symptoms of energy blocks, where the current is short-circuited and broken down. This is called "disease" named after the structure plus 'itis' (inflammation) or 'algia' (pain), such as appendicitis, neuralgia or a complete breakdown 'lysis,' like in paralysis.

There are over fifteen hundred diseases, and only the transgression of Nature is the cause of most of them. Therefore, by removing the cause, a multitude of symptoms will disappear. Hence, keeping the skin active, as well as internal cleanliness and natural food which can be digested, are great factors in maintaining health and balance with Nature.

When ill, in pain or in fever, give the body a rest from food and simply drink hot water with lime, lemon, or grapefruit juice in it, for a few days, until you feel better. "Starve a cold LEST you feed a fever" is an old slogan and a good one to follow. Animals do all this naturally and instinctively, but man is ignorant of Nature's simple way.

Baths: A warm bath in the morning is very good. For this bath use a wash cloth with soap on it and also some baking soda (soda bicarb) and table salt on the soapy cloth. Mix two parts of soda with one of the salt (not in the water but dry on the wash cloth that is wet and soapy). This should be used on the face, neck and all over the body. It is a cleansing and refreshing bath, and has the soothing effect of bathing in the ocean. Such a bath removes the gummy substance from the pores and eliminates body odor. Then rinse well with warm water and use cold water, especially down the spine, as a final shower. This closes the pores and one does not catch cold after the bath. Even though there is no danger of this in the summer time, a cold rinse is always refreshing and invigorating. While the body is still wet, rub the entire body, including the face, with olive or almond oil, or some good body oil. It takes very little to cover the entire body—by first blending a small amount in the wet hands, then rubbing them over the face, arms, legs and body. This dissolves certain types of gummy substances on the skin, which water and soap will not remove. Then briskly rub the body dry with a towel. In fact, the body will be practically dry by then, but a brisk rub with the bath towel is also beneficial. The body will then feel refreshed and cleaner than ever before.

People with LOW BLOOD PRESSURE, poor circulation and low right pulse should not take full hot baths. They need cold water as one stream down the spine, to tone the capillaries and the vasoconstrictor muscles, which control them. Repeat this cold water application several times, for ten seconds each, at the end of a warm bath, as described above under "Baths."

People with HIGH BLOOD PRESSURE: Hot water applications and baths are for high blood pressure and for pains, spasms, and for dilating tense capillaries. A hot sitz bath for pains in the lower back is a good relief measure. Always follow this with a general quick cold shower to close the pores, plus the oil rub while the body is still wet. To curl up in the tub with hot water covering the torso, legs resting out on the tub, gives one a good sweat, and may be taken for ten minutes or so, then shower off and follow up with the oil rub. This is a good daily health measure and is very refreshing.

The foregoing, in brief, is a simple routine to regain health. Stretching, mild exercise, deep breathing and walking are also very helpful. (See Part II of this volume.)

Sex and Emotional Balance

Sex indulgence, like alcohol, temporarily gives a false sense of elation, which is inevitably followed by a state of depression, because the cerebrospinal fluidic essence, which is the conductor of the highest Vital Energy in the body, is expended. The presence of this Energy Essence is necessary in every cell of the body, for rebuilding and repair, healing and constant replacement of new cells for old worn out cells. Cellular vigor and function depend on this Primary Life Energy. In fact, over-indulgence through any of the senses leads to mental as well as physical illness, exhaustion and depletion.

Such impulses cannot be conquered permanently by mere suppression but only by supplanting them with desires and impulses of a higher order. As long as unfulfilled desires of any of the five senses are lurking in the mind, there is frustration, and frustration leads to ill health. Emotions are the inner chemistry of life.

The only desire that truly can be fulfilled for all eternity and which has only good consequences, is the longing for conscious union with God, which union is known as "God-Realization." Any effort made in that direction invokes His Grace to enable us to make more effort, until the Goal is reached. This can be achieved only under the guidance—and protection—of a Teacher who has himself travelled the Path.

That is the very purpose for which we have been given this human form. It is the temple of God, made by God Himself, and in which He resides and can be realized. It is up to us to use it as a means to fulfill that purpose. With that object in mind, we should try to keep this body in a fit condition—mentally, emotionally, physically and spiritually.

Thought and Action

Besides diet, right thinking and right living play an important role in the state of our health. Equilibrium, as balanced energy flow, is the secret of well-being.

We are Physical Matter and have a physical body:
What we eat and drink,
*   we become physically.*

We are Emotion and have an emotional body:
What we feel and sense,
*   we are emotionally.*

We are Mind and have a mental body:
What we think and dwell upon,
*   we are mentally.*

But our soul Consciousness is a spark of the Supreme Being, which can mold life to any pattern and being, into any state of becoming, by effort, by love and devotion to Reality, the Oneness in all life. However, this cannot be realized universally until we have realized it within ourselves. And for that we need the guidance of One who has achieved God-Realization and can give us the Key. By giving up the ego-consciousness, we may enter the consciousness of Eternal Oneness, by His Grace.

The Creator is one! His life is the core of all Being, Consciousness and Bliss—the Essence of Oneness. Soul is a child of the Eternal Father and needs a True Guide of the Inner Life to regain its lost estate of Conscious Bliss, which enfolds all.

LOVE'S TRAPPINGS

When Love was trapped,
Into forms unwrapped,
It declared each one,
A vestal virgin of the Sun.

The beams of light,
Shone fresh and bright,
Enraptured with delight,
In the moonbeams of the night.

This pristine glory of the Sun
Was bestowed on all and one,
Who fell in love with Love
Lost to earth and Heaven above.

7

Polarity Function in Man & the Universe

"Health is the proper relationship between the microcosm, which is man, and the macrocosm, which is the universe. Disease is a disruption of this relationship."

— Dr. Yeshi Donden, physician to the Dalai Lama

All matter, emotions, mind substance and energies move by the three modalities of 0 (neuter), + (positive) and - (negative) polarity. These were called the three gunas, or the three mountains or prominences in the mind region of Trikuti: Mount Meru or Maru in the center, Sumeru on one side and Kailash on the other.* This is the cosmic picture of energy modality, demonstrated by the orbits of planets around a central sun.

The microcosmic picture we find in the atom and in the cell: A nucleus or neutron in the center, which is the Satguna type energy; the Rajaguna energy, which is a positive centrifugal energy of heat and expansion, flying upward and to the right, repelling in its red fiery nature of the sun; the Tamas energy, called the moon energy, which is a negative centripetal energy of moisture (like a precipitate of the positive pole), settling downward and to the left. [Tamas is the attractive power of the negative pole of energy emanation, the moon-type energy of cooling, green rays—the feminine precipitating, centralizing, toning and quieting principle, the nest-building instinct in all living things, which becomes resistant to change.]

---

* These are all symbols derived from Hindu cosmology.

The atom and the cell are bipolar in their function and energy whirls of circuits. Positive and negative charges dance around a nucleus or neutron charge, like a central shaft or dividing line as we find it in the cell (♈) dividing the right from the left. It is the astrological sign of Aries, finished in its lower half of the negative sphere of precipitation.

COMPOSITE PICTURE OF THE PATTERN FORCES
OF THE BODY AND THEIR WIRELESS CIRCUITS.

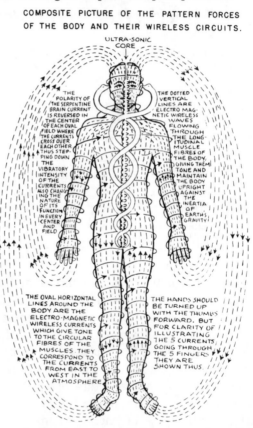

The central, Satva guna or Satguna neuter pole is the axle around which all these energies revolve. This describes the ancient swastika in its whirling motion, like a spinning fiery disc, called a chakra by the ancients. All centers of motion

*The above diagram of basic energy flow is taken from Chart 3 of Dr. Stone's *The Wireless Anatomy of Man.*

are such spinning discs of energy, as wheels of light and fiery motion. According to the Bible, Ezekiel saw the same by the River of Life as the expression of energy, which he called the Chariot of the Lord of Life. He said it was a "wheel within a wheel" (like the atom).

The human body is a magnified cell, the expansion of the brain pattern of the airy neuter, all-present Life Energy Principle, which has its base in the cerebrospinal fluid—in the brain and in the spinal cord and throughout the entire nervous system. The middle of the human body is the neuter pole— from the top of the head down through the spinal cord and its three coverings. The cerebrospinal fluid flows between the pia mater and the arachnoid sheets, and follows the nerves all through the body. The right side of the body and the right side of the head is the positive pole. It gives off positive energy currents. The left side of the body and of the brain is the negative pole, and radiates negative energy currents. This knowledge and awareness can be used by every person to balance his or her own energies and thus relieve pain.

Pain Relief Through One's Own Polarity Currents

An excess amount of the positive current produces irritation, pain, swelling and heat in the tissues, organs and areas of the body, due to excess amount of blood in that area, and the opposite or negative pole energy is required to balance it. The positive current is the sun energy of fire and radiant warmth in normal amounts. *The right hand* is the conductor of this energy. For negative tension, congestion, spasm and stasis, the right hand contains the antidote, the positive polarity current. Place it over the negative symptoms for relief.

The left hand is the conductor of the negative or moon current, which is cooling, soothing, refreshing and toning. Place it over the seat of pain, where the positive currents are in excess, giving the symptoms mentioned above. Wherever the pain is, that excess calls for release of the irritation, heat and swelling, which the negative current can provide.

The positive or right hand is placed opposite the negative. If the pain is in front, place the left hand over it, and the right hand on the same area on the back, to get a current through the congestion. If the pain and the congestion is on the side, place the left hand over that area, and the right hand opposite, on the other side. If the pain is on the top of the head, place the left hand there and the right hand below it, on the back of the head, or under the jaw if the pain is nearer to the front than the back.

If the pain is in the spine, you can use either the flat of the left hand, or double the hand up into a fist, and lie on it, wherever the pain may be located, so as to get the pressure along with the application, as both are indicated. This is done easily by lying on the back in bed or even on the floor. Then the right hand is used over the abdomen, directly opposite to the left hand in back. Hold this position for ten or fifteen minutes, and changes will take place in the electromagnetic fields of that area and bring relief. This is the most potent remedy, ever present in the hour of need, which can be used by every person on himself or herself.

Cold water and hot applications constitute a thermal remedy, to change the circulation locally and to increase the capillary circulation. Hot applications increase the circulation and dilate, by bringing the blood to the surface. Cold applications tone over-dilation, constrict the circulation and contract by driving the blood into the deeper structure. This thermal expansion and contraction is not the primary energy current and it is not as effective as the use of the hands. The right hand generates heat and the left hand is cooling.

Gentle stroking with the left hand has a very soothing, sedative effect. With the right hand it is stimulating. For the same reason, downward stroking is soothing, while upward stroking—from the feet up to the head—is stimulating. This can be done with both hands, because the direction determines the polarity here.

The front of the body is sensory and receptive, and attracts. The back of the body is motor and repelling. For example, to turn our back on a person is to slight or dismiss him. Sensory pains have their origin in front of the body. Motor pains are usually of the bones or muscles and are found in the back.

All polarization is done from the front to the back, from side to side, and from the above to the below, or the superior to the inferior. What healing power lies in the hands of all beings, for themselves and for others, has to be tried to be convinced by proof. It is the primal electromagnetic energy of the molecular construction of the body. It is not a mystery, nor supernatural, any more than the principle of expansion and contraction. The nerve currents are the same energy in a conducted form for specific impulses from one definite area to another. The nerves act as wires. The molecular structural energy is wireless, but is tapped by switches in the brain, to flow over definite regions, and nowhere else. Polarity Therapy is a precise localization of currents for definite functions in the body.

The Creator gave each person energy, which flows from center to circumference and returns by polarity action. It also flows from within outward, and from the top downward, and returns by reaction or attraction from the surface to the center and from below to the above. That is how life works and the motor energy goes out, and the senses report back the result of the outgoing experience. By these paths of energy or light waves and rays, we can reach cause and effects in the body, and balance them within ourselves by mind and emotional polarity or balance; and with the hands, as energy polarity of the pranas or the five life breaths which animate the five senses, as sensory and motor functions.

According to the Bible, the Lord said to Job: "Then will I also confess unto thee that thine own right hand can save thee." (Job 40:14)

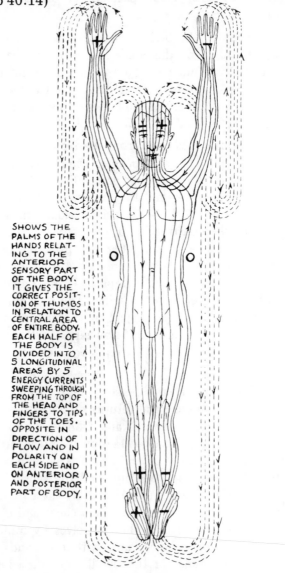

SHOWS THE PALMS OF THE HANDS RELATING TO THE ANTERIOR SENSORY PART OF THE BODY. IT GIVES THE CORRECT POSITION OF THUMBS IN RELATION TO CENTRAL AREA OF ENTIRE BODY. EACH HALF OF THE BODY IS DIVIDED INTO 5 LONGITUDINAL AREAS BY 5 ENERGY CURRENTS SWEEPING THROUGH FROM THE TOP OF THE HEAD AND FINGERS TO TIPS OF THE TOES. OPPOSITE IN DIRECTION OF FLOW AND IN POLARITY ON EACH SIDE AND ON ANTERIOR AND POSTERIOR PART OF BODY.

*The above diagram showing some of the basic positive and negative currents is taken from Chart 6 of Dr. Stone's *The Wireless Anatomy of Man*. Note the right hand's positive, outflowing energy and the left hand's negative, inflowing energy as described in this chapter.

8

Live Food without Killing

*"Explanation is for the Mind;
Inspiration and Vision are for the Soul."*

When a lion makes a kill and eats part of the warm animal, he is getting as close to live food as he can, but he is eating a carcass just the same, whether it is freshly killed or the next day or after that. The lion is carnivorous by nature, whereas man is herbivorous, as evidenced by the teeth and the digestive system. Yet the lion has an instinct which directs him to the vital organs of his prey, to eat them first in order to get the precious enzymes, hormones, vitamins and minerals in them. This is the process by which the carnivore gets his supply of enzymes, hormones and other essentials besides bulk food. Man buys cod liver oil or shark liver oil for its high vitamin A content. The lion eats the raw liver and gets the same benefit. Instead of obtaining vitamin A and the other vitamins and minerals from animal sources, mankind would benefit much more by getting them from plant life, the way the Creator intended. We find evidence of this in the Bible and in the teachings of all the Great Saints and Sages.

Right now, while I am writing this in America, I am vacationing on a lake in the north woods of Wisconsin. There are bear, wolves, foxes, deer, chipmunks, gophers and other types of wild life in the woods. Some of them come shyly to the cabin now and then. Mice and bats are the real problem, as they will get into the house occasionally. I have observed that the mice will carry away cherry pits and eat out the kernel, after which the pit looks like a bead with only one small hole in it. They will also carry away watermelon seeds and eat out the center, thus getting the vitamin and enzyme values that they need. The chipmunks will gather the wild cherries and do the same. They will also eat almonds and other nuts out of our hands, and become real friendly. Who taught them these secrets, that "the Life is in the seed"?

And man, in all his cleverness and by improper use of mind and intellect, kills this life in the seed or discards it and looks for remedies elsewhere to sustain himself and fill in the missing link with gross chemistry and its complexities. Man eats for pleasure, and the animals eat to survive in Nature. Anyone can sprout grains and other edible seeds in the house all year round and can always obtain some fresh greens for chlorophyll or even expose the sprouts to indirect sunlight for the last two hours of their growth, to make them green at the finish.

These are not secrets but mere observations in Nature, which is so richly endowed with life and shared by all her creatures who live in her domain and chirp a song of praise to the All-wise Creator. If we are in tune with the Inner Life, we are automatically in harmony with Nature and its energy currents.

A Simple Live Diet

A simple live diet which includes all the value of the lime and lemon and the oil with garlic in it, as well as the various sprouts and lettuce or fresh spinach and cucumbers or carrots and fresh, tender young peas, uncooked, is to make a meal of these items and to eat them as a salad with a dressing of the oil and lemon or lime, with the addition of honey to taste. A salad of this type, eaten with some burned toast for its charcoal value to sweeten the stomach, is a complete meal.

Thus one can get all the values mentioned and necessary for human nutrition, in a single meal which is energizing, refreshing and not stuffy or fermentive. Even a meat-eating person will tell you that he feels lighter and brighter after such a meal than he does after his heavy meat and egg meals. If one desires some cooked vegetable dish, the sprouts can also be added to that when it is served, but not during the cooking process.

Even the lion or tiger cannot get all these values in his fresh kill. The fresh sprouts, fresh greens and drinks made from them, and the fresh fruits make up a natural diet for a thinking person with a vision and not merely an appetite to satisfy. Once we experience and realize this, we are no longer satisfied with "dead food," nor do we crave it, but rather prefer the natural and nourishing foods which are even less expensive and no fuel is required for their preparation.

We must live up to an ideal or purpose to fulfill our life and grow in Love and understanding, which the Creator gives to all His children, out of His bounty and grace. When that is our objective and viewpoint, then Devotion and Gratitude fill our life and we are happy.

9

A Nutritious Diet for Rich & Poor Alike

"Too much education—
not enough understanding!"

An adequate and nutritious diet is the big problem in life, not only where there are so many poor people but also in countries with plenty of food, like in America. An inadequate diet is not always due to not being able to afford the proper food but to improper selection of what is available. And, strange as it may seem, the best food is not always the most expensive food.

Merely eating plenty of rich food is not the answer to health nor to well-being, nor to a good physique. Food that is too rich clogs the cells and overburdens them in their function of digestion, assimilation, elimination and oxidation. Poor health is more often the result of excessive intake of food rather than a lack of it. Hungry people are usually more healthy and active and have more children than the wealthy, well-fed people. In the light of this understanding, the poor need not be envious of the rich, because their very poverty is a protection for them from the excessive intake of rich food and the resultant ill health which would be theirs if abundance was their lot.

The problem which most nations have with feeding the poor is not so impossible as it looks. We are always poorer in vision and understanding than in food and the necessities of life, because if we have the vision and the faith in the Creator, and work with understanding, the necessities would always be provided. In the Bible, Proverbs 29:18, we find that

Solomon the Wise King said: "Where there is no vision, the people perish."

Now let us see how this works out in life and how the poor could be better fed, with the things they already have and which are easily obtainable, and with greater economy, if used wisely. We all know that poor people cannot afford to buy fresh citrus fruits, tomatoes, etc. to get the necessary amount of vitamin C, although there are some fruits which cost little.

But the facts are that only one-half cup of soy bean sprouts contains an amount of vitamin C equal to *six* glasses of orange juice. While any of the grains and legumes are suitable for sprouting, the simple and easily available alfalfa seed is considered the best of all as it contains all the known vitamins, including K and B_8; besides potassium, often called the Elixir of Life; phosphorus, which is considered good brain food; and calcium, so essential for bones, teeth and general well-being. The necessary chlorophyll can be obtained by exposing the sprouts to indirect sunlight during the last two hours of their growth, but better still, from other edible green leaves and grasses, either as fresh salads or made into a drink, as previously described, and taken with lemon, grapefruit, lime or pineapple juice. That is not only curative, nutritious and prophylactic, but delicious as well.

One cup of soy beans or alfalfa seeds, or foenugreek or other seeds will yield up to ten times its bulk in sprouts and will nourish a larger number of people than if that particular cup of beans, peas, or other seeds were cooked, and will provide a greater amount of vitamins, proteins and minerals than the cooked food. If, as a matter of habit, one wishes to eat some cooked food along with this, one may do so, but it is not necessary. The lack of good nourishment is a lack of vision and the knowledge to use what we have with understanding and appreciation of its value.

Grains are usually available to the poor and are often given to them by the government for food and for seed. If not, then wheat, oats, rye, barley, millet, corn, soy beans, mung beans, garbanzos, foenugreek or alfalfa seeds are usually reasonably priced and easily obtainable. All these seeds have life locked within them, which can be turned loose by means of a combination of moisture and warmth.

This sprouting process is not a secret, but the mystery of the life value and all the nutriments in those sprouts, attracted from the universal energy fields, are a wonderful means to better living and good health. Why not use these living foods?

Due to lack of vision and understanding, the very poor and the rich alike will grind up the grain and cook the legumes, and thus kill the life principle in them by heat, without ever unlocking the secret "Open Sesame" of Life in them through the process of sprouting. One can even cook the sprouts to better advantage than the seeds themselves, but it is essential that some or most of the sprouts are eaten fresh rather than heated or cooked.

In this connection one must not overlook the fact that "well-being" does not mean merely a well-nourished body, for then man would be no more than a contented animal. Our attitude and the thoughts we think are even more important than the food we eat, and for proper guidance along this line we need a spiritual teacher.

10

Limes & Lemons as Home Remedies

"I go with what nature verifies."

Limes and lemons are so much alike that we speak of them as having the same value. Most citrus fruits (limes, lemons, grapefruit and oranges) aid oxidation and elimination by the stored-up airy energy in their air-tight compartments. Vitamin C and calcium are their main contributions as food values. The lime and the lemon are particularly valuable for these factors, plus the new vitamin P which is found in them.

The airy element in this citrus fruit is so active that its uses and benefits are limitless when used with understanding. Limes and lemons play an important part in aiding digestion of protein foods, especially when used in combination with fresh papaya. Citrus fruit also changes the over-acid condition of the body to an alkaline one by its heavy fruit calcium contents, which supply the bones, teeth, blood and nervous system with calcium and phosphorous.

Because of this, these citrus juices are a great aid to *nervous persons*, and are used in *neurasthenia* with fine results. Citrus juices relieve and prevent *nervous indigestion* and *halitosis* (bad breath) due to upset digestion. Actors and business and professional people find the lime and lemon a great help to keep their breath sweet by drinking the juice of either, sweetened with honey and diluted with water, before or between meals and before retiring. This is also good for *sore throats* and *colds*, especially if pineapple juice is added to it. Lemon or lime juice is a great remedy for *asthma*, by using

67

two tablespoonfuls before each meal and before retiring—in addition to a starch-free and milk-free diet.

Lemon juice also has an antiseptic value and a healing and dissolving effect on abnormal tissues. When mixed with almond or olive oil, it is a wonderful remedy for *eczema*, applied externally and used internally as well. In bad cases of *eczema*, use a starchless, all fruit diet, including the lemon and oil internally and apply the lemon and fresh pineapple juice externally every hour until cured.

Athlete's foot yields quickly to the application of lemon juice, especially when combined with fresh papaya juice. The dissolving effect of lemon juice has been shown also in *cataracts*, by putting several drops of a solution made up of equal parts of lemon juice and distilled water in the affected eye or eyes three times daily.

For *pyorrhea*, a combination of lemon juice and table salt rubbed into the gums several times daily has given excellent results after other remedies had failed. This also cleanses and whitens discoloured teeth. *Felons* are dissolved by inserting the inflamed finger or toe into a half of a lemon over night and cleaning it up in the morning.

Erysipelas, considered a highly infectious disease, yields nicely to lemon juice compresses, and is healed in this simple way after all the drugs have failed to give relief.

Coughs and *colds* are helped by lemon juice, especially when mixed with honey, some garlic and fresh pineapple juice. If the fresh pineapple juice is not available, the canned will do. The mixture is even effective without the pineapple juice, but the addition of the pineapple juice yields quicker results. This is a wonderful remedy even in *diphtheria* and other throat conditions. For *diphtheria* the lemons can also be roasted until they crack open, then extract the juice and mix it with the above ingredients to dissolve the stringy mucous in the throat so that it can be expectorated by the patient. It would also be helpful for the patient to gargle some of this mixture every hour or so, until relieved. In *biliousness, influenza, jaundice,* and the after effects of *over-indulgence,* (*hangover,* whether from too much food or drink) there is nothing like lemon juice and a fruit diet to clear it up.

Alcoholism and the *tobacco habit* can be overcome easily, by sucking a lemon whenever the desire to indulge is active. This is not only a perfect substitute but is also a builder and replacer of the lost phosphates, calcium and vitamins needed to balance the system. Abstinence from meat, fish, eggs and heavily spiced foods, as well as maintaining a rational nourishing diet, must accompany the cure. Any determined patient can be cured by this method in a month or more.

For *wrinkles* and *lines under the eyes* there is nothing better than a mixture of lemon juice and olive or almond oil, gently massaged from under the outer corner of the eye, inward, toward the nose; also, from the same outer corner of the eye in an upward diagonal direction. This same mixture is also excellent for the scalp and for treating any scalp infection.

To keep *joints* and *feet* pliant, especially for dancers and artists, there is nothing better than to rub them with equal parts of oil and lemon juice.

For *rheumatism* and *arthritis,* use the morning liver-flush daily. This has been mentioned in previous chapters: or take the juice of half a lemon before each meal and before retiring and adhere to a strictly vegetarian, non-starch diet for this condition.

In *chills, fever, headaches,* use the fresh lemon with clover or alfalfa tea freely and abstain from food until these symptoms disappear.

For *dropsy* and *cirrhosis* of the *liver,* peel the lemon, cut it up, cover it with honey and eat it. Start with one lemon a day and go as high as ten a day by adding one each day, until improved then work backwards down to one a day. One should remain on a fruit and juice diet while on this procedure.

For *fatigue* and *thirst quenching*, the lemon and alfalfa tea is good. Or suck a lemon when exhausted or thirsty. It is far better than the vinegar and water drink used for that purpose in hot climates.

Diarrhea—whether the patient is young or old—can be overcome by the use of apple pulp mixed with lemon juice and a little honey and powdered cinnamon sprinkled on the mixture.

For *piles*, go on a fruit and vegetable diet, taking no water. One-half cupful of warm olive, cotton seed or suitable vegetable oil, mixed with one-half cupful of strained lemon juice, should be injected into the rectum at night and retained over night or as long as possible. The patient can wear a pad and protect the mattress with a rubber or plastic sheet.

To reduce *swelling*, whether it is of the throat or enlarged breasts, use lemon juice compresses. For the compresses, one may dilute the lemon juice with equal parts of cold water.

In *cosmetics* and *beauty* treatment, the lemon is of great value, whether it be for a hair rinse, for reducing enlarged pores or for whitening and softening the skin. It is of great help in removing *objectionable odors* from the hands such as after peeling onions or garlic, and is also a stain remover, for such as fruit stains. For the hands, simply take the rind of the lemon after the juice has been squeezed out and rub the fingers and hands with the remaining pulp.

Lemon and oil sniffed up through the nose is a great cleanser of the *nasal passages*. This will also clear up *adenoids*.

For *constipation* take a mixture of half a cupful of lemon juice with half a cupful of olive, almond or sesame oil four times a day, until the bowels move.

For *poultices* on *boils*, *abscesses* and *skin eruptions*, apply the pulp of the lemon, and take the juice with the oil internally also.

As a *gargle* for *sore throat*, use lemon and oil, and take it internally also.

For *vaginal hygiene* and *leucorrhea,* lemon juice in water, in varying amounts, will be most helpful to relaxed or irritated tissue.

The skin of the lemon is a flavour delicacy. Grated or chopped fine, it can be added to salads, baked goods, and puddings. Even marmalade is made from the citrus fruits. Some seagoing veterans have even used marmalade made from lemon or orange to counteract *seasickness.*

Moth repellent—Use ripe lemons into which cloves have been stuck to make them look like brown balls of cloves. Put them around in clothes closets and in the pockets of the clothes. They will dry and leave a fine fragrance as well as prevent the moths from getting near them.

Please note: Wherever almond oil is not available, olive oil or sesame seed oil will do nicely when it is to be taken by mouth; otherwise, even cotton seed oil or other vegetable oils may be substituted for external use and for the rectal injection. Only in cases of *severe enteritis* and *colitis* is the healing effect of the almond oil preferred, along with the lemon, as a treatment.

11

Mineral Value in Foods

"Only God and nature cures."

Minerals are essential to keep our chemistry in balance and to supply our bones, blood and tissues with the elements necessary for normal function and growth. Dr. Julius Hensel called attention to this fact long ago, when he wrote his book, *Bread from Stones*. He was the first pioneer in this field and, as an expert chemist, he laid a good chemical foundation for nutritionists and doctors to follow. Later, the Biochemic remedies of Dr. Schussler followed the same pattern in the Homeopathic field.

To give just one explanation and example of Dr. Hensel's philosophy and application of mineral value in the lymph stream, he quoted the terrible epidemic of smallpox in northern Canada, which wiped out whole villages in the spring of the year. The cause was the lack of minerals in the bloodstream, because of a lack of foods which contain them. Dr. Hensel said that the excessive use of meat and white flour combinations was the cause of this disease, which implies that the diet was lacking in the necessary vitamins and minerals.

In smallpox, the lymph gets so thick that it cannot flow, because of the lack of minerals needed for its circulation. Iron is necessary in the bloodstream to enable it to convey oxygen to the tissues, and this cannot be done without the iron in the red cells. As a result, the thick lymph is pushed out as pox, and the disease is called smallpox.

Minerals are needed in the tissues for tone and as conductors of electromagnetic light waves, which link the chromosomes of the cells to the finer energies of Nature. Without these basic conductors, the molecular energy has no field in which to operate. The quality of tissue and its elasticity depends upon the full nourishment needed by the cell and supplied by the foods that are alive with vitamins, enzymes and minerals as well as proteins, starches, sweets and fats, besides the bulk. These may or may not contain what the cells need in energy-conducting factors or mineral building blocks.

All vegetables and fruits are rich in minerals, as are grasses and grains, when properly prepared as food. The juices of vegetables and fruits have been used as juice-therapy, for better health, by many ailing persons as well as by healthy people to maintain good health. The juices are extracted from fresh fruits and vegetables, and used at once so that they do not oxidize and ferment when exposed to air.

Nature puts a vacuum seal in all her fruits and juices in the fibres of the fruits and vegetables. To extract this by crushing the fibres, makes that juice available in its natural state, with all its mineral contents, and has proven most helpful to many run-down constitutions when other means had failed. It is a means of simple health-building with better building blocks than were used before.

Fresh celery juice is rich in sodium and has many uses. It is one of the best vegetables for juicing as it covers so many of the body's needs. It also has a pleasant flavour and is helpful to the nerves and a good night's sleep if taken before retiring.

Carrots are rich in natural vitamin A and are used most freely by juice advocates, in combination with celery, cabbage, parsley, beets, kale, string beans, brussels sprouts, spinach, or any one of the green vegetables. Even garlic has been used with some of these vegetable juices, especially for high blood pressure.

For *diabetes*, carrot, celery, string beans and brussels sprouts have been employed successfully as a juice, used daily, by sipping about a glassful three times daily. The juices of *beets*, *parsley* and *watercress* are very concentrated and should *not* be used *too freely*. About four ounces per day, mixed with other juices, is plenty.

For *asthma, bronchitis* and all *catarrhal conditions*, carrot and radish juice has been recommended as well as total abstinence from cream, ice cream, starches, sugars and eggs. And to open up the sinuses and air passages, use horseradish and lemon juice. Grate four ounces of horseradish, and two ounces of lemon juice, one teaspoonful of garlic juice and one tablespoonful of honey. Mix and take a teaspoonful or more of this mixture four times daily.

Sesame seed makes a very fine drink when ground fine and mixed with water, with a little honey and lemon added. Sesame seed contains vitamin T, which is a new discovery for prevention of internal bleeding of capillaries. During the War it was discovered that the Turkish flyers had superior eyesight, which was traced to their extensive use of "Tahini," the name given to finely ground, hulled sesame seed. Although it is classed with the "fiery" foods, it does not cause or irritate piles as is commonly supposed. The Turkish flyers did not find it so. Improved oxidation is the real factor here, under the Fire Principle, rather than an internal heating effect which Ayurved* has taught. The new discovery of vitamin T proves this fact in the sesame seed, which has a tonic effect on capillaries and vessels to *stop the bleeding*.

When raw potatoes or mushrooms are added to the raw alfalfa sprouts, the combination makes a complete food for enzyme, vitamin and mineral content. That is a perfect food in all elements needed for health. Even *tuberculosis* has been arrested by the use of raw potato juice. Grate the potatoes or put them through a juicer, allow the starch to settle, then pour off the juice. Combine one-half glass of this clear juice with one-half glass of raw carrot juice. To this add a teaspoonful of

---

*Ayurved: An ancient healing art of India, several thousand years old and still extensively practiced today.

olive or almond oil and a teaspoonful or so of honey. Beat this until it foams; drink three glassfuls of this mixture daily and eat plenty of alfalfa and foenugreek seed sprouts every day.

In *stomach* and *intestinal ulcers,* a combination of carrot and cabbage juice is used daily, plus the sesame seed drink previously mentioned.

For *nervous conditions, neurasthenia,* and for cerebral tension of *epilepsy,* celery, carrot and lettuce juice is used freely—three or more glassfuls daily.

For *varicose veins,* carrot, spinach and turnip juice is recommended.

For *low blood pressure,* carrot, beet and dandelion juice is used.

For *gall bladder* trouble and *gall stones,* as well as *kidney stones,* carrot, beet and cucumber juice is taken.

For *constipation:* A combination of cabbage, spinach, celery and lemon juice.

For *skin conditions, boils, pimples, carbuncles:* Carrot, beet and celery juice.

Arthritis: Carrot, celery and cabbage.

Anaemia: Carrot, dandelion, parsley, spinach and beets.

Adenoids and *tonsils:* Carrot, beet and tomato juice.

Poor circulation and *heart:* The juice of carrots and beets.

Goiter: A combination of carrot and watercress juice.

Gastritis (inflammation of the stomach): Carrot, celery and cabbage juice.

Hemorrhoids: Carrot and parsley juice.

High blood pressure and *phlebitis* (inflammation of a vein): Celery, beet and carrot juice.

In using greens for juices for their mineral and vitamin contents as fresh building blocks for the system, one must make sure that none of these greens are sprayed for insects or disease. Whenever sprays have been used on the greens, that makes them totally unfit for juice and as a food. Very few persons can tolerate food that has been sprayed with insecticides, and food that has been contaminated by these sprays cannot be recommended. The only other alternative is the sprouts, which you can raise yourself and know that they are not sprayed.

12

The Mystery of Sprouts

"Energy flows through matter and animates
it. Otherwise, matter is as dead as a doornail."

Seeds contain a hidden life principle as well as a moderate amount of vitamins, enzymes and minerals. But in the process of sprouting, all this is increased tremendously. By subjecting the seed to warmth (the fire principle) and moisture (the water element), the life process is set into motion. Thus the electromagnetic light waves are attracted from the etheric tattwas (elements), which bring with them the other elements needed for growth. This energy-condensation of light waves attracts the necessary vitamins and determines the pH of the cellular activity. High condensation makes for acidity, and low for alkalinity of the cellular chemistry.

But here is the mystery of increase: there is practically no vitamin C in dry seeds; however, tests have revealed that when the sprouts first began to peep out of soy beans, they tested 108 milligrams vitamin C; and by the end of 72 hours from the time they were first soaked, they contained 706 milligrams of vitamin C! So the beans and any other edible seeds that are used for sprouting, contain the highest amount of C within a period of 72 hours from the beginning of the process. It is therefore suggested that the best time to eat them is between 60 and 80 hours from the time of soaking them. After that, the vitamin C content begins to drop off, as it is used for the development of the plant's growth. They should be eaten then or put in covered glass jars and kept in the refrigerator until they can be served in salads, soups and other foods, for the vitamin values as well as the proteins and minerals which they contain.

Other vitamins also were found to increase in the sprouts. Vitamin B_1 and Pantothenic acid doubled in the sprouting process. Biotin and Pyrodoxine were increased about 150%. B_2 and Folic acid increased by nearly 500%. Two doctors at the President College in Calcutta found the important constituent, Choline, climbed 20 and 30% respectively in black-eyed peas and wheat, during four days of the sprouting process. The vitamin E in mung beans was found to increase by one-third, in the same length of time. U.S. Experimental Feeding Stations found that by feeding five pounds daily, of sprouted oats, to breeding animals of both sexes, their fertility was increased, and even confirmed failures were restored to usefulness.

When beans that are used for cooking or baking are sprouted beforehand, their nourishing quality is greatly increased and their explosive nature is quietened—a most useful factor where excess gas (wind) is the problem. It has also been found that by sprouting, much of the original starch contents are converted into simple sugars. This gives quick energy, as the monosaccharides enter the bloodstream almost at once, without requiring any digestive changes, and thus eliminating the subsequent letdown of energy. Alfalfa sprouts have 150% more protein than wheat, oats, or corn. The chlorophyll contents can be increased by putting the finished sprouts into indirect sunlight for two or three hours.

Good, wholesome nourishment, with high vitamin and enzyme contents, is thus available to all seekers after health and better living, with just a little thought and care in preparing sprouts from grains and pulses that would ordinarily be cooked or baked without these added hidden values.

13

Principles of Good Digestion

"Fear and desire are the two things that rule us. Now, how much of a Master are we of those two things?"

There are a few essential points on the principles of digestion that blend with Nature's process so smoothly that mankind has overlooked them completely, although all herbivorous creatures observe them naturally. Man is the highest form of creation and his digestive tract is designed for a herbivorous diet.

THE FIRST PRINCIPLE is the thorough chewing of starches in the *dry* form, to mix the starch molecules with the saliva and with the enzyme ptyalin, to start the digestive process *in the mouth*, while breaking up the fibrous envelopes or coverings of the grasses and grains by means of this thorough mastication and insalivation. Every cow and buffalo follows that naturally, by instinct. They can even bring up their cud and chew it over, because they have a storage stomach for that purpose and they are not in a hurry.

If the starches are ground-up cereals that are cooked, such as oatmeal, cream of wheat, and other breakfast cereals, then the saliva cannot penetrate the molecules of the starch thoroughly because they are already fully saturated with moisture in the cooking process. Even insalivating them then does not penetrate the saturated particles to mix the enzyme

---

*This chapter was originally written for inclusion in the Urdu edition, published in India in 1970.

with the starch molecules. And dry, prepared breakfast foods, such as corn flakes, wheat flakes or puffed rice, are usually drenched with hot or cold milk or cream, plus sugar or syrup. This also saturates the flakes and leaves no room for the saliva to make direct contact with the starch molecules, which need to be broken up by the saliva to enable digestion to take place.

The sad part of it is that this well-established breakfast habit everywhere, supposedly for the sake of health, has caused so many ills to the human race that it is hard to believe, until it is traced through thousands of cases of indigestion and its train of illness that follows. The aftereffects of this type of breakfast have been a big headache to many physicians and patients. *Diabetes* is only one of the many consequences of the inability of the body chemistry (of the pancreas) to digest the starches that were unprepared by the saliva in the mouth, plus the addition of white sugar taken daily. The artificial sweeteners are even more detrimental to health.

In children, such breakfasts as mentioned above have caused all sorts of catarrhal and mucous symptoms of the throat, nose and sinus congestion, as well as tonsilitis, adenoids, eye and ear trouble, and susceptibility to colds. We often wonder why children should be so subject to these ailments as a general rule, when the young animals living in Nature do not have these ailments.

For over fifty years I have searched for an answer to this problem in a busy practice until I found that even adult indigestion is rarely diagnosed, properly treated or relieved in general practice all over the world. This came as a shock to me when I was consulted by patients of wealth and means who had traveled to a dozen or more countries in the world in their official capacity and who had sought the answer to their health problems from eminent practitioners in those countries, but found no relief. By the Grace of God I was able to help them when all other methods had failed. We can easily brush this off and say that the general public's habits cannot be wrong; but they suffer just the same. What needless suffering, when the cause can be pinpointed and solved!

Therefore, I repeat the key principle: Starches should be chewed *dry* and not washed down with liquids, such as milk, coffee, tea, soups or water and other beverages. Chewing and insalivation *is a must* for the enzyme's action in all herbivorous creatures and starch eaters.

Many sick persons got well when they started *Fletcherizing* their food (the process of lengthy and thorough mastication and insalivation of food in the mouth) and *eating less.* Dr. Fletcher discovered this simple fact many years ago when he was very ill, and the proof was a healthy life after that. Hence, the name of "Fletcherizing" was given to this process of thorough and lengthy mastication and insalivation. His book on "Fletcherizing" is well known.

Rice is a starch and when cooked properly, as it is in the Orient, so that every kernel is whole and dry, it is a well-established diet of millions. Poor people enjoy it and chew it well when they have so little of it, and they stay well. Some author in Japan even recommended rice as a cure-all, without stating the real fact behind it; namely, a mono diet* and thorough mastication. This, of course, applied to the natural, unpolished rice from which the valuable rice bran has not been removed.

Plain potatoes, boiled with the skins on them, served a similar need in early Pomeranian Germany. This was the main diet of the peasantry. They ate these potatoes only with soured skim milk (curd), and they did not know what illness was, due to this simple mono diet, which included whole-grain dark bread without butter. They performed hard physical labor and so this diet was suited to their circumstances; but for sedentary workers potatoes may be a bit too heavy. Here I

---

*Mono diet: A diet which consists of a single kind of food.

merely want to point out that it is the *simple diet* and one *suited to the individual needs* that is essential for health.

Dr. Metchnikoff called the world's attention to the Bulgarian peasants' acidophilus or yogurt diet years ago. But when taken with all the rich foods, it causes fermentation and acid reaction in the system. Acidophilus and yogurt stands or booths were quite a fad in the French Riviera some years ago; but the fad ceased when rheumatism set in due to this fermentation. An excess amount of lactic acid is one cause of sore joints and muscles. I have had numerous cases where their illnesses were the result of this acidophilus or yogurt idea having been overdone or carried to the extreme. In order to be beneficial, the acidophilus or yogurt should be taken in small quantities and *only when it is fresh*, as it reverts to plain lactic acid within twenty-four hours after it is made.

THE SECOND PRINCIPLE is that *protein foods are digested entirely by the enzymes in the hydrochloric acid in the stomach.* That is why protein foods should be eaten first when they are a part of the meal. This enables the proteins of peas, beans, lentils, cheese, etc. to swim in the juice in the stomach and become saturated with it, before all the other foods or drinks dilute this enzyme mixture of hydrochloric acid in the stomach. That is why it is a good policy not to drink with meals, and especially *not cold drinks*, as these lower the temperature at which digestion takes place in the stomach. Rich protein foods with fat in them can cause a real upset when a cold drink is taken with the meal. Cold drinks taken with a meal of animal protein can cause a serious illness afterwards—even more so than when the protein is a vegetable derivative.

I do not recommend high protein diets and concentrated foods such as brewers' yeast or fresh yeast. It is too clogging and upsets the vitamin balance in the body. In fact, I have found it necessary to take many patients off of this course of concentrated and artificial selections of supplements. This fad of a high protein diet is often the cause of illness, and when the high protein is of an animal nature, such as flesh foods and eggs, the consequences are even more serious.

Not only have I found this to be so in my practice, but eminent authorities, such as W. C. Rose of the University of Illinois, say that we need less than twenty-five grams of protein per day. Other leading nutritionists have also found that one can get sufficient protein on a diet of fruit alone if supplied in suitable quantities and varieties. All these well-known authorities also state that the high protein diet has been greatly over-emphasized and has done much harm. This is especially true when the protein consists of flesh or eggs and their derivatives. The "hidden hunger" is not caused by a lack of food or lack of protein, but by a *lack of proper nutrition.*

THE THIRD PRINCIPLE is that only foods that are properly digested are useful to the body in its chemistry of replacing worn out tissue cells, minerals, vitamins and enzymes. Foods that are natural and have the power of growth in them are the richest and of the greatest value in the "pranic" energy of the sun, which also produces the chlorophyll in green leaves, fruits and grasses that are so nourishing to man and beast. Greater selection of these varieties gives more *vital energy replacement,* plus their mineral and vitamin content, than the concentrated proteins, cooked foods and chemically prepared substitutes and supplements. These facts have been well covered in other chapters of this book, including the value of sprouts as living foods.

Fried foods are almost indigestible on account of the welding job between the foods and the fats under high cooking temperatures. Such foods are injurious to the liver and the kidneys, and often produce liver symptoms and yellow jaundice. Also, cooking foods the usual way and adding oil or butter to the food in the cooking process does similar damage in a lesser degree and leads to indigestion—pains in the *calves of the legs, arms, chest* or the *back muscles.* Why cook fats into the food at all? Why not add them when serving the food, so the high temperature of cooking won't weld them together and make them indigestible? Do the same as when we add oil and lemon to the salads as a dressing. *That is digestible!*

THE BREAKFAST PROBLEM: A heavy breakfast in the morning is a big mistake in the economy of the body's chemistry, because all the tubes and their mucous linings are in a state of rest and repair during sleep, exchanging secretions of their cellular tissues in a relaxed state of rest. So they *need flushing out in the morning,* the same as we wash out the mouth and brush the tongue and teeth with some cleanser, which gives that refreshing feeling.

The herb teas recommended earlier, as well as lemon or lime juice in hot water, are of great service and do an excellent job of flushing these tissue cells. Fruit juices made of grapefruit, pomegranate or oranges, or a combination of them, are very good. Even plain hot water and honey is very good. To this one may also add any of the citrus juices. One can also make a healthful fruit drink by combining the juices (*always freshly made*) of apples, carrots, edible greens, zucchini and other fruits or vegetables in season with the addition of *fresh* fruits and/or vegetables. Oranges, grapefruit, papaya, pomegranate, any melons in season, apples, pears, peaches, plums, berries—whatever is desirable and in season—are the fresh fruit selections needed for breakfast to give the body chemistry its much-needed "prana" (life-breath) in these vital and natural foods, with their sealed-in juices. In other words, it is best to remain strictly on the above mentioned liquids and fresh, juicy fruits and vegetables during the entire morning. Then the body is prepared with a natural appetite for a good meal at noon.

Here it seems well worth repeating that only the food which is properly digested and distributed in the body is useful and health-building. Carburetion in a motor and its oxidation of fuel is a similar process to digestion in the body. Like carbonization in an engine, congestion in the body is due to indigestion and results in many symptoms and ills. Stagnation invites fermentation and breeds bacteria.

The mood that we are in when we partake of food and drink has a great bearing on the digestive system. The best food is indigestible if taken when one is in a state of anger, tension or too much excitement. At such times it is advisable to partake of warm liquids only. Of course, the best remedy is not to get into such a state in the first place; but if and when it does happen, we only add insult to injury by loading the stomach with a heavy meal.

Results in health or the reactions of indigestion, which can be checked at various body points—even pains in the hands, arms, shoulders and feet, as well as the local discomfort over the stomach and liver and intestines—tell a real story that cannot be denied. Causes produce effects, and symptoms of pain so often are caused by indigestion. Removing the real cause of distress will cure the ailment and the symptoms.

PHILOSOPHICAL OBSERVATIONS: The flow of the "prana" currents in the body is the same as the energy of the sun acting in Nature as a whole and is needed by every cell for its function and life in the human body. This "prana" function is the real physiology, because it supports all sensory and motor functions in the body. "Prana" is the river of life, as the vital current of the body, in its five-fold action. It is the distributor of the Life Force (the vibratory sound current from the *Anahad Shabd*,* the non-vibratory Sound, the Tree of Life) throughout the body.

The "tattwas" (elements of earth, water, fire or warmth, air and ether) are the fields and structural tissues of anatomy. They support the "life winds" of "prana" that flow through

---

*Anahad Shabd: Also called in Western traditions "The Lost Chord," "The Word of God," or the *Logos*.

the house we live in and call our body, the temple of Being on this earth. The human body is a rare gift from the Creator Himself and should be understood and treated intelligently.

Liberation is not for all souls at once; it is the consciousness itself that must grow up out of the childhood state of toys and possessions and their experience of action and reaction through pleasure and pain, that souls eventually learn the celestial refrain, as the true balance of freedom from pain.

Correction of causes is not for everybody, as that spoils the illusion of suffering; they would much rather have their ego massaged and indulge a little longer in their self-limited estate, rather than learn the essential Truths of Life from Nature and from God. The body is a part of Nature and must be tuned into Nature's rhythm of finer, subtle energy-flow, as cells breathe the air, which in and out does go.

14

A Purifying Diet
An Effective Purifying and Reducing Diet, Especially for the Chronically Ill, Based Upon Over 60 Years of Practice & Research

"Man is ill because he is never still."
—Paracelsus (Often quoted by Dr. Stone)

The following Purifying Diet should be taken as long as there is constipation, high blood pressure, arthritis, rheumatism, pain, swelling, congestion, toxicity, and overweight.

MORNING TIME is used for flushing the system and cleansing it. No solids are taken—only liquids, including plenty of fresh grapefruit, oranges and lemon juice; or fresh grape juice in season; but *no* milk, regular tea or coffee. It is most important to flush out the liver, the kidneys and the intestinal tract in this way, to restore their correct chemical function. The entire well-being of the body depends on this.

Instead of bed tea in the morning, take two or more cupfuls of hot herb tea made of Licorice Root, Himalayan Mountain Violet, Anise or Fennel, Peppermint, and Foenugreek, to which should be added at the time of serving: fresh lemon juice, fresh ginger juice to suit the taste, and honey if desired; but sugar should never be used. Several glassfuls of this may be taken at a time during the morning between meals, or any other time—day or night, as desired. If constipated, use more licorice root and fresh garlic. In diarrhoea, use no licorice, ginger or liver-flush, but substitute cinnamon bark in the tea and use powdered or finely ground cinnamon with baked apples and/or dates and raisins, chewed thoroughly. Blackberry juice relieves it at once. Cinnamon, cooked with rice and barley water, or barley and curd are also effective in diarrhoea.

NOTE: A good quality of *cold-pressed oil* with lemon is a cleanser for the liver, while cooked or fried oils or fats of any kind are bad for the liver and will clog it, especially when the fats are cooked or fried into the foods at a high temperature, which then cannot be separated and digested at the inner body temperature of 105 degrees.

FOR BREAKFAST: Take from three to four tablespoonfuls of pure, cold-pressed almond, olive or sesame seed oil with twice the amount of fresh lemon juice and add fresh ginger juice to taste. This I call the "liver-flush." If you can get grapefruit, add the juice of one grapefruit or several oranges, and drink it. Chew and swallow three to six small cloves of garlic with the oil mixture. Then have the hot tea mentioned above without sweetening. That is a cleansing breakfast, which helps to oxidize the tissues. Do not use honey with the liver-flush.

NOTE: The seeds from the lemons, grapefruit and oranges can be chewed and kept in the mouth for fifteen minutes or more, after breakfast or any time that the citrus fruit is taken, to get the benefit of the enzymes, vitamins and minerals which are locked up in the seeds. This bitter essence is also good for the liver and gallbladder. Even the white coating, just under the rind of the citrus fruits ought to be chewed, as that is also beneficial, for it contains citrus bioflavonoids, an essential vitamin C factor. The oils contained in the outer portion of the rind are a bit too strong to be chewed and may be harmful to the enamel of the teeth. Every portion of the citrus fruit can be used, with the exception of the outer oily rind, which may be grated off and used for flavoring fruit drinks, other dishes and salads. In such minute quantities it is also very beneficial.

The seeds should be chewed thoroughly, and then the residue can be spit out. This is a valuable procedure, which adds to the vital benefit of the fruits as cleansers and utilizes the whole fruit. Nothing is wasted in this way. Chewing these seeds after taking the garlic removes the odor and taste of garlic, as does also chewing some parsley or other edible greens of high chlorophyll (green) content. Brushing the teeth with a good toothpaste also helps to remove the garlic odor as does chewing fresh mint leaves, or cardamom or cloves and the like.

TWO HOURS AFTER BREAKFAST: Have eight ounces or more of fresh vegetable juice made from green cabbage, carrots, lettuce and other edible greens that are available, along with one or two ounces of red beet juice. To this may also be added the juice of radish, onion or turnips to suit the taste. Also, ginger juice, fresh lemon and honey may be added, if desired, to suit the taste. Two or three cloves of garlic may also be chewed and swallowed with this drink.

NOTE: Sip this juice slowly and thoroughly insalivate it before swallowing to obtain the greatest benefit from it. In fact, all foods should be thoroughly masticated and insalivated before swallowing to enhance digestion; and the insalivation also applies to the liquids. Liquids are taken between meals by themselves, not with meals.

NO OTHER FOOD should be taken with this morning cleansing diet, and that means positively *NO* toast or starches of any kind. This diet is for the purpose of cleaning out the souring process of digestion and its gases, which give rise to all kinds of symptoms and gas pressures that resemble heart pains. Fermentation of souring food is the cause of arthritis, rheumatism and many other ailments. The body must get rid of these sour ferments, sedimentations and gases somehow in order to be well, as they are the background of pain symptoms and illness stored up in the tissues of the body over long periods of time. That all has to be resolved in the healing crisis of elimination, like dirt is pounded out of laundry. Only clean fabrics, clean body tissues, take on the color or dye of health. The liver-flush in the morning with fruit or vegetable juices, a raw salad with a baked vegetable dish at noon, and fruit for supper is an ideal and simple diet for health.

AT NOON: Take a raw salad made of fresh greens, like lettuce, finely grated cabbage or other edible greens in season, together with grated carrots, radishes, turnips, sliced cucumbers, tomatoes, green onions or whatever is suitable and available. The contents can be suited to taste, but should definitely include sprouts made of mung or soy beans, foenugreek and alfalfa seeds. To this salad may be added a dressing of almond, olive, sesame or other good vegetable oil together with lemon and ginger, garlic, and onion to suit the taste. If there is constipation, then add some pears to the salad. A pomegranate, papaya, mango, apple, pear, grapes, figs, dates, or raisins—any one of them or a combination makes a nice dessert. This constitutes a delightfully wholesome meal, providing all the necessary protein, vitamins and minerals in an appetizing and easily assimilable form, as found in Nature. A dish of plain baked vegetables, with sprouts and lentils may be added if hungry.

NOTE: Boil for about one hour, the vegetable pulp residue from the vegetable juice made in the morning, together with onion, if desired; strain, and take this as a hot beverage between meals. Add fresh ginger juice to suit the taste; a little black pepper can also be added to vegetables like cabbage, cauliflower and turnips to prevent gas formation.

During the afternoon take another glass full of fresh raw vegetable juice, like in the morning. Again boil the residue vegetable pulp, to which other fresh green vegetables or leaves may be added as desired and available, which can be used as a hot soup later in the afternoon or before retiring. Fresh fruit juices can be taken between meals or at night, but not with meals.

EVENING MEAL, DINNER: Use papaya freely, or fruits like apples, pears, grapes, and pomegranates plus the herb tea as a beverage. Or, if very hungry, repeat the noon meal of salad, especially the sprouts. Proteins and fruits are a good combination at one meal. When the health improves, a little more food is permissible. Food must be digested to be nourishing.

NOTE: From this it is quite obvious that *no* milk, butter, coffee or regular tea is to be taken, as well as *NO* potatoes, rice, bread—*NO* cereal products of any kind and no sugar, and definitely NOTHING FRIED. Just one piece of bread or toast would be enough to nullify the otherwise good results of this diet, because of starch fermentation.

Also please note that *no* aluminum cooking or serving utensils are to be used, as that also would counteract the good effects of the diet and is definitely harmful.

BATHS: Take a warm tub bath, and on cold mornings a hot one, sufficiently hot to perspire for about fifteen minutes. Soap a wet wash cloth well and on it sprinkle about one tablespoonful of baking soda (soda bi carb) and use it on the face and entire body to cleanse and open the pores of the skin and thus remove the sticky oil which causes body odors. Then rinse with warm water and get right out of the tub and under a cold shower for about fifteen minutes, with all the pressure possible, direct from the pipe, after removing the spray head from the pipe. Let the water run full pressure, well up and down the spine and shoulders and all over the abdomen, rubbing and slapping the skin at the same time to activate it.

FLUSHING OUT THE COLON is also very important, and for this an ordinary shower hose, with the spray removed, can be used to conduct the cold running water into the rectum, while squatting; expel immediately and repeat this until the expelled water is clear. The effect in the colon is a refreshing rinse. One feels clean and refreshed all over. The water is not retained, but run in and out quickly to bring down the debris by a natural action. In cold climates the water can be tempered or used quickly.

NOTE: If you will follow the entire routine strictly, without consulting your own opinions, habits and appetites, you will notice improvements that will astonish you. If you want to follow your own inclinations or habits, why consult a doctor?

A Word About Sprouts

Sprouts can be made from any edible seed—Nature's own laboratory—in a simple way, in one's own home, by spending only a few minutes each day. Sprouting increases the natural protein, enzyme and mineral value of seeds, by the special germinating process, which opens up Nature's hidden values of the secret caves of living energies in all seeds.

We all need fresh enzymes, vitamins and minerals which Nature uses to build her own realm, to feed man and beast alike. Anyone can do this sprouting of seeds or raising of wheat grass like flowers by imitating Nature and then combining the results (sprouts) or wheat grass in a tasty dish, by adding them to any salad or serving them plain and fresh along with some cooked vegetable or soup, or even with fruit. They are good for all persons—well or sick. *The sick are in greater need of them,* as they lack these finer energies of Nature, which is the reason for their sickness. It is the finer tissues and nerves that need this living energy and enzymes set free by sprouting, to rebuild health in the most economical way. Nature knows best. It is her real medicine and food combined into her master building process of rejuvenation by liberating the energies. Anyone looking for health should not neglect this vital process of Nature. Chewing them well *is the patient's essential business* in order to obtain all the finer values plus the manifold increase in bulk of the finest quality. Another method is to plant wheat in boxes, and cut the grass for salads and eating raw when about four inches high. This is the best healthful green available and can be raised at any time.

A NEW AND EASY WAY OF MAKING SPROUTS requires several large-mouthed jars, into which the hand can easily be inserted several times a day to wash the slime off of them, then rinse with plenty of fresh water and drain off the water, so that they do not sour.

First, soak the required amount of seeds—one-half to a cupful at a time, depending on how many people in the family are using them. One-half cupful of seeds should be washed in warm water and then covered with plenty of warm water— two to four cupfuls or more, as the seeds will expand over night. Keep the jar covered with a cloth or simply a brown paper bag or newspaper and preferably in a warm (not hot) place. In the morning pour off the water, rinse the seeds thoroughly and add no water, but drain off the excess so that the seeds are merely moist but not standing in water. If the weather is hot, this has to be done about three times daily; if the weather is cool, once a day is sufficient, and the jar may be placed—covered to keep it dark—in the sun to keep it warm. The seeds need warmth, moisture and darkness and to be kept clean by rinsing as mentioned, and they usually mature, ready for use, in about three to four days. After that they can be used and the remainder stored in a glass jar in the refrigerator for daily use, and a new batch started so that it will be ready by the time the first one is used up. An easy way to drain off the excess moisture after rinsing the seeds and later the sprouts, is to place a strainer or cloth over the mouth of the jar and turning it upside down until all the excess moisture has drained off. Once the sprouts have matured and are stored in the refrigerator, they need no further care. They can best be stored for several days in a covered glass jar, from which they should be used.

Alfalfa sprouts are considered the king of sprouts, and especially good for rheumatic and arthritic conditions. Foenugreek sprouts are soothing, healing and at the same time dissolve the gummy substance from the mucous membranes and intestinal lining, and enable the system to absorb the benefits of the intake. Sometimes one can take the best of foods and beverages, but when the linings are so thickly coated with this sticky substance, one does not receive the benefit, and this is where the Foenugreek is of great help. The mung or mung bean as well as the soy beans are rich in protein and are tasty builders of tissues and energy.

This getting-well process is a serious and earnest business, which requires the *best attention of the patient's mind and will* to do what is necessary to eliminate the toxins, wastes and ferments from the body, which are the cause of disease. Even if one is under-weight, the body cannot absorb the nutrition and increase in weight until all these waste products are eliminated from the system.

Our body is our house and temple in which our soul lives as consciousness and king in its own domain. It is our responsibility, and no one else's, to keep our temple fit and clean and well. Self-pity and crying over illness is no solution at all; but finding out the cause and eliminating those bad habits (such as smoking, drinking, excess of or too rich or fried foods, or being a slave to appetites and sense pleasures—all of which weaken the natural reserve energies) is the patient's first business, duty and responsibility in order to get well and stay well. The no-breakfast plan with only the liver-flush and fruit juices is most helpful by itself, to get well and stay fit.

A person must be well to do his or her best and fulfill one's hopes, aspirations and destiny in life. Are we willing to keep our "temple" fit for the Master's visit within our hearts? Effort and diligence is the price of HEALTH AND HAPPINESS.

Exercise

Patients constantly ask for an exercise to keep fit. The simple answer is, any exercise is good which keeps the shoulders free and movable, and assists in respiration and digestion. The muscle which is located over the shoulders on each side and down to the middle of the back controls many digestive reflexes, which should be kept free to function properly.

A simple and easy exercise would be to sit on the side of the bed or a chair and place both hands on the chair, outside of the knees, and bend forward as far as it is comfortable. Then, with your hands braced thus, push the body upward and backward with your hands, to *lift the body back into the straight, sitting posture.* You will then feel this freeing movement between the shoulders and the back, which relieves that tension and weariness at once. Do this for about five minutes, any time when you are sitting down. It will surprise you by its effective helpfulness and relief of shoulder tension, pain and gases. This is an unusually simple and efficient exercise for anyone. It is so easy to do at any time or place. Asthmatics get great relief from it. This exercise is illustrated in Part II.

The subject of exercise can be elucidated by an explanation of certain primary energy principles, and Part II of this book does just that and also illustrates many simple and easy exercises that have a remarkable vitalizing effect.

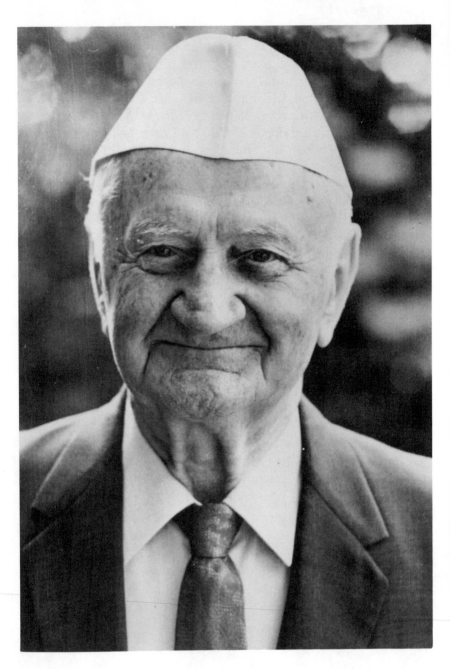

Dr. Stone in India.

Part II

Easy Stretching Postures for Vitality and Beauty

Based on the natural position of the
body during the period of gestation
for most favorable results in
maintaining and repairing the
energy current flow —
the primal factor in health and beauty

Introduction to
Easy Stretching Postures

Presented herein is a quick and efficient method of self-help for solving the many problems of health encountered by everyone, young and old. Especially very busy men and women will find this shortcut to well-being a great and useful boon. It requires only a few minutes anywhere in private to practice the postures explained in this book.

The Wireless Energy Currents of Polarity in the body are beneficially affected as one gently and gracefully wiggles into the postures. The squatting position brings the three airy energy fields, one immediately over the other, into active and reactive tension flow of energy waves. The idea itself is an "Acre of Diamonds" in everyone's own back yard, previously totally overlooked. We can deal with vital atomic energy in ourselves *right now*, for pain and tension relief as well as for steady improvement in our health.

To assure the good reader that these seemingly difficult postures can be mastered and that much benefit can be gained by regularly and consistently following these principles and practices for a few minutes each day, please allow the author to make the following statements:

All that is offered herein is based upon personal experience and facts worked out by practice. The principles used are the same as those given by the author in his books entitled *Energy: The Vital Polarity in the Healing Art, The Wireless Anatomy of Man*, and *Polarity Therapy*,* explaining the concept of finer energy currents in Nature and in man's body—reciprocal and interchangeable in essence—upon which depend our lives and health here on earth.

The author passed his 64th birthday on February 26, 1954.† He had not been able to correctly take these postures until the discovery of the gentle rocking motion to shift the polarity constantly from one group of muscles to another, which made the accomplishment of the postures possible.

Within three weeks after this discovery and the application of the principle of "effortless effort" in this posture work, the author was not only able to pose for the illustrations presented in this book but also was able to hold them all the while they were being sketched.

The idea of a youthful life at 65 is not too farfetched when it can be demonstrated!

Sincerely,
Randolph Stone

---

*All three of these books, as well as others by Dr. Stone, are available from CRCS Publications (address on title page).

†Dr. Stone lived an active life for almost 30 years after he wrote these words and he continued to use and teach these postures. In addition, Chapter 23 includes material that he published in 1970 on other exercises that he developed in later years, most of which were a further development of the original exercises that he first publicized in 1954 in a small booklet.

15

Latent Energy Fields in the Body

"When the energy currents are out of balance, we experience physical, mental and emotional symptoms of discomfort, pain and sickness. Shorts in energy circuits in the body must be found and re-established. . . . Man has a wireless energy arrangement similar to that of the atom and the universe."

The popular concept of exercise is muscular exertion to increase the circulation. But there is something finer which floats like an etheric essence of energy in the blood and which may be called vital energy, life energy, or the spark of life. Even the Bible states that the life of man is in the blood. The old Hebrew Scriptures called it "Ruach" or spirit of life. A great mystery resides in this fluid medium known as the blood stream.

To get new blood to the tissues is the purpose of all exercise, massage and gymnastics of various types. In 1909 Dr. August Bier of Berlin, Germany formulated and published his famous textbook on Hyperaemia. He said, "Give more fresh blood to any part of the body and it will heal." Upon this principle many therapies were founded, such as use of suction cups, steam baths, electric cabinets, percussion massage, etc.

Breathing exercises and lung expansion had this principle in mind also, by getting more fresh air into the lungs and to all the tissues. The modern administration of oxygen has the same purpose, without the strenuous exertion which is not for sick people. However, before the oxygen can take its place in the tissues, the carbon dioxide and waste gases must first be eliminated because they are chemically opposed to the function of oxygen.

When the pelvis is right, everything in the foundation of the body structure is right. When the vital energy currents roll naturally in their orbits, there will be less tension, frustration, emotional upsets and restlessness. Many emotional and mental conditions could be benefited by these simple basic relaxation exercises. No force is ever used. All that is required is a gentle coaxing of the mind and emotions along with the muscles and the posture. It is not the accomplishment of the posture which is important, but the *energy current flow* which is established as a result of the posture. It is not the perspiration—which is merely the effect—but the relaxation and the natural tone gained by the gentle exertion that really matters.

This new principle of exercise (energy-current-release by posture-stretch-relaxation) is a more natural aid to health than all the forceful muscle straining used in many other methods. Athletes do not lengthen their span of life, but rather shorten it by heart strain and hardening of muscles all over, which in turn throws more strain on the central pump. Statistics prove this from sad experience. For example, Frank Gotch, the outstanding wrestler of his time, died at 42 years of age.

Posture is the simple way of nature, which moves the inner machinery of life's forces and leaves the muscles as elastic as a kitten's. The posture stretch gives more pliability to the fibers and spring to the step, more color to the cheeks and luster to the eyes. "Not by force nor by might, but by my Grace, saith the Lord."

The age of muscular power is fast passing by, due to the advent of all our modern conveniences and the mechanical leverage of machinery. Might is by mind and atom power now, not by muscle and brawn. In these days things are accomplished by inspiration and integrity around a central principle, not by perspiration. Not by number, but by skill and good will does man accomplish. Brute force is gradually losing out everywhere. It no longer appeals to the youth of this age nor to the female of the specie as an outstanding accomplishment. Agility and health, yes; but not bulk in appearance. Dexterity of mind and thought go much better with an elastic body than a rigid one. Nature proves that. And a nimble wit rarely goes with a rigid type of body which has been subjected to much strain.

For the tense businessmen and women, posture stretches used during office hours would pay well when the mind sags and gas problems bother and interfere with the mental work at hand. A walk would take more time and not accomplish this much current flow, providing the new blood supply to the head and flush to the cheeks. And strange as it may seem, it is not done by standing on the head nor by aiding gravity nor by pushing the circulation around by force. Neither is it done by forceful breath control. In this work no breathing exercise is needed except as a stretch of muscles, by expanding the chest cavity with a natural deep breath and exhaling with a grunt that vibrates the tissues.

When the breath is used in a posture, it is for a general stretch of the tissues from within, outward, in order to *reverse* the day-long routine of constant impacts from without, pushing inward. No wonder we often feel like violence when the outer impacts become too forceful and continuous. Try this posture for a safety valve and benefit by the astonishing results.

Many mysteries are locked in the brain of man, the observer and thinker, the positive pole of the body. How many such secrets of equal importance are locked up in the pelvis, the negative pole? Have we ever asked ourselves this question? In proportion to external scientific pursuits, how much attention has been given to man himself? Experience teaches that man's growth and *real* life is an individual problem. And it must be so in order to leave him a free agent. Life is an expression of the soul of man from within, outward. When he succeeds too well in the outer, he usually forgets the inner Source of life altogether until illness or other misfortune strikes.

Is it not possible for man to keep well by doing a few simple things daily and living less strenuously? The answer is yes. In the pelvis, the negative pole of the body where all the driving force is pent up like a coiled spring, a release needs to be found which equalizes this tension *without force or waste of vital energy*. The downward eliminative functions of Nature must be stimulated in order to give clearance for the currents' return to the head, the positive pole.

Vital force has its base in the sacrum, which is the motor force in the pelvis. The rest of the body can share this vitality only if its currents are flowing over the body in normal circuits of finer energy waves. If it is wasted or blocked in its circulation, the body's entire vital economy suffers and ill health is the result! Vital force is the motor and elixir of life for which there is no substitute anywhere. There are millions of seekers like Ponce de Leon, but the answer remains hidden from external search alone.

A house rests on its foundation. So does the structure of life in both man and woman rest on the vital force located at the base of the body, the pelvis. Its tissues are vital, and even the bony structure and articulations are fundamentally important for all motion, action and well-being. Many ills and pains which are the despair of physicians originate in the pelvis. Just mention a sacroiliac lesion, a lower back pain or sciatica, and few insurance companies will accept the risk or continue to provide health coverage.

Yet how much time or attention or effort of inquiry do we give this vital subject of our life? How much time are we willing to give it now, regularly, when we have found a way to gain daily benefits and improve our health? Only a few minutes several times a day are needed, but *regularly!* It is not an easy posture for Westerners to take, although it is in everyday use in the Orient. And because it has been so thoroughly neglected, the need is even greater and the results are truly astonishing. It is a challenge to our integrity to keep well and to make a regular effort in assisting Nature to do so. If external cleanliness is said to be next to Godliness, what could real *internal* cleanliness accomplish, plus the improved energy flow of the life forces which must reach the brain for its vital function?

The negative pole does support the positive, even as woman sustains man in his finer emotional life and creativeness. Without that there would be no creation or even mental brilliance or inspiration from life's Source within. The latent energy fields in the body present a definite and new approach to the problem of the circulation of the energies in the body, conducted or wireless, which are essential to our well-being.

The body as a whole consists of two opposite ends and a middle, which are polarity fields with polarity functions, relationships and subdivisions. Zone Therapy in its field of amazing reactions could never be explained otherwise and make sense. If the good Doctor Fitzgerald had known this scientific fact behind the marvelous results he obtained, Zone Therapy would rank among the accepted discoveries in the healing arts of today. But for lack of a true principle as a foundation, a fine art was lost to the majority of the profession, and its benefits were lost to the public. Opposite poles are fields over which energy travels and functions. Electricity, chemistry and the magnetic field prove it as a purely practical science now. But to extend that idea to other living fields and functions has found little favor in the healing art for the benefit of man.

To link posture or exercise to the energy fields in the body and their functional improvement is a new and startling idea within the Western healing arts that I have presented in the book, *The Wireless Anatomy of Man*. The foundation is laid, which may be accepted many years hence as a fact and a part of the healing arts. However, those who are interested may prove it to themselves NOW in this simple application of a posture-stretch which is unique in its effect, and sound in the deeper principles of life and energy-flow. There must be pioneers for every new idea, or our world would stagnate and become utterly uninteresting.

There are primal pattern energies and fields in our make-up, which are as true and essential to our function and life as a blueprint is to a well laid out structure or a mechanical design. These pattern energies are a fine, wireless variety of the nature of mind substance and emotions in their various step-down functions as currents and waves. *These patterns are the designs and the unseen builders in our body and in Nature everywhere.* The original pattern in God's design is in the seed power of each thing according to its kind. The neutron entity is the hidden factor in each field around which these particles of matter spin by an attractive, innate, individual force of their own. Each unit and specie attracts and builds its form according to its pattern and the kind of energy latent within it. This throws some light on the mysterious creation of our body as a polarity function.

These finer energies laid out the pattern fields by their spinning polarity functions, and the keynote of the pitch of their vibratory particles attracted to each center of action. It was such a process which laid down the intricate brain tissues and nerves, as wires for conducted nerve energy and more detailed specific functions of the human body, and also the miles and miles of arteries, capillaries, veins, lymph vessels, and ductless glands. This energy not only builds the polarity fields, but also *is* the energy which flows in these conducted conveyors which maintain the body and its functions.

Having introduced a foundation for this principle in active operation in our body (as the electromagnetic motivator over polarized fields), let us see how we can apply it and benefit by this new discovery of Nature's wireless forces. The posture is an approximation of energy fields, which brings positive and negative poles closer together, causing an energy flow—not enough to make sparks fly, but so the average person can feel a favorable reaction of some kind after making even a few efforts to take the postures. This will differ with each individual, as some are far more sensitive than others. But the eventual results are certain as the polarities act and react on each other in fields and centers of function. Gravity and pressure are merely external aids for conditioning, but they are not the real factors moving the main currents of the body; they only assist the solids and gases in their motion of elimination.

The postures are given in easy steps, so the process is a natural, progressive approach without force. The postures are designed and used as an easy way of *effortless effort*, to move the deeper energy currents of the body by a process called "Wu-Wei" in the East. This literally means "doing by not doing." Let Mother Nature do it by co-operating with her and resting on her bosom. Thus let the Universal Currents take over the job. It is literally riding the River of Life's energy waves and tuning into them! It rests upon the understanding of Nature's law and the polarity of posture—positions—of the body. And these postures are not based on the erectness of the body to defy gravity. It is an effortless way of merely placing the body in a tension field where the airy energy principles are gently stimulated, so the vital forces can flow freely through the body and its muscular tissues, giving it more elasticity and a greater freedom of function through polarity balance.

Even as planetary bodies exert an influence in certain relationships to each other, so do their representative electromagnetic fields in the human body stimulate or inhibit vital function in that individual. That is why we feel better when the sun is shining brightly and on certain days when external vibratory magnetic stimulation gives us a lift. Science has proved that sun spots have a definite reaction on life and the well-being of mankind, and that the position of the moon has a definite relationship to vegetation and the sea. Judging by these effects in Nature in general, man cannot be isolated or left out of the beneficent and alternating action of the Universal Energy Currents.

A seed, planted in the ground, does nothing of itself. It is merely positioned into a natural environment where it can sprout by the action of forces from the outside. *Then* it liberates its potential energy which was dormant, and its own centrifugal and centripetal pattern forces express themselves in Nature's embrace of the good mother earth. Energy can lie dormant in a seed for centuries, as was proven by kernels of corn found in the hand of an Egyptian mummy which grew when planted. *How many latent energy fields, of both physical and spiritual possibilities, lie dormant in man!* The physical benefit is our main consideration here. THE FINER POSSI-BILITIES AWAKEN WHEN THE INDIVIDUAL IS READY!

The main postures in this book look very much alike, but each stimulates different energy fields. The basic squat has as its objective the stimulation of the air currents in the body, especially the downward function of the current flow which tends to all the natural elimination. Then, when the outlets are open and the drag and resistance is released in the negative pole, there will be better positive intake of air and oxygen. The result is improved neuter pole action, distribution of energy, oxygen and food supply through absorption and better assimilation of it in the blood stream and in the tissues.

This is accomplished by placing the body *in an exact position of all three airy energy fields, one above the other*, where each is stimulated by the other pole in its field. The most negative is released first, which makes room for the action of the others. It is as simple a matter as when a plug is pulled out of the bottom of a barrel, the liquid will flow. But this liquid acted upon is an energy current which is regulated from a latent center of finer polarity forces *in the body*, not dependent on the gravity of the earth. Gravity will assist only in the expulsion of the solids and liquids of elimination. The posture is ideal for that purpose. It is natural. But the actual currents started in this process are the finer, individual energy waves which are more or less inactive in their response to the energy fields outside. The cerebro-spinal fluid is the medium for conduction of this finer energy in the body—over the brain, the spinal cord and the nerves which are its physical conductors.

When the body energy does not flow with the rhythm of its source of supply, it is out of tune and cannot obtain the "broadcast" of Nature for its own radio-active functions in its field of operation. This idea may present a new view on the energy flow of the individual life with that of Nature, which is its reservoir. When that exchange ceases, the airy principle which was the life of matter goes back to dust. The fires of life become ashes, and the earth goes back to the earthy elements of Nature to be reassembled into other units of living structures with individual energy centers and active fields.

Movement & Physical Health

Nearly all the primitive races knew the secret of agility which lay buried in the pelvis. The South Sea Islanders and the Hawaiians, who have fine physiques and graceful carriage, kept themselves so by their dances of free hip movement. Whether we call them belly dances or "suggestive" does not matter. These rhythmic movements together with a contented mind kept the islanders agile, alert, free and happy in their mental outlook and in their work, which was more like play.

If we worked as hard at attaining perfection in hip movement as they did from childhood, we would forget our superficial comments on appearances and instead value the results gained in health. Let anyone study ballet dancing and they will soon learn what it takes to do a few simple steps in rhythmic motion. Even as the pelvis is the water basin designed by Nature to give birth to new life, it is also the source of energy to *regenerate* the existing life and recharge its fields.

Exercises should be rolling and rhythmic, using life's other wise dormant field and its latent forces in the pelvis to develop and keep the body young and agile. Combined with song and dance, the mind and emotions are also employed in rhythmic exercise and the routine is forgotten. This type of exercise can be likened to a turbine engine in action. The Western nations have over-emphasized the mere physical exertion of muscles against resistance, which is like the piston engine. The compulsion of hard work and military stress and training have always overdeveloped the purely physical aspect of forceful motions, which travel like a piston in a cylinder. It brings out the hardness and compulsion of civilization.

We admire the free grace and natural elastic carriage of the South Sea Islanders. This is their heritage through song and dance in rhythmic motions, which were ceremonial as well as festive. Some of their devotion was also expressed in dances, which was a new idea to the suppressed white man. The natives had but few problems in morals until the white man came along. Each tribe had its own rules and standards which were strictly observed, and the punishment for violating them was not less severe.

Other races of the East, who did not have the easy life and the customs of the South Sea Islanders and who had less time for song and dance, developed postures to accomplish all that and more! In the absence of chairs and other comforts, Nature favors the squatting posture. It is natural all over the East, especially in India. Statistics show that 70% of the population of the earth use the squatting posture.

Rhythmic expressions of song and dance, which use all the bodily forces and muscles for expression, free the emotions by naturally liberating the energy blocks, suppressions, frustrations and stagnations. And when mind, body and emotions are used in one effort of rhythmic exercise, it becomes a triune health movement of balance. This same effect may be produced by taking the simple squatting postures illustrated in this book. These postures favor the control of the mind by balancing the energy currents and producing quiescence or mental peace.

16
The Purpose of the Postures & Why They Work

"Energy itself has intelligence which must have a direction of flow or a way to go, or it defeats itself in useless expenditure and destruction. Every energy block in mind, emotion and in matter is an obstacle which often necessitates eruptions of a volcanic type in Nature, and disease in man and beast or in vegetation. In such conditions the norm of the mental pattern of energy flow, in form and use, has been interrupted and must right itself. The wise man and physician looks for the cause and assists Nature in balancing this directional energy circuit back to its norm— physically, mentally and emotionally."

In the macrocosm, the constellations and stars embody keynotes of atomic forces which differ in polarity and effect. This causes an influence and a reaction when they come into proximity with other orbs. In this world's system, with the sun and its radiations as the central orbit, sunspots have a decided effect on everything that lives, grows and moves. The moon and the other planets also have their radiation and influence on each other and on individual life, whether human, animal or vegetable. These effects have been charted and worked out into very complicated details and systems by astrology and other observations.

When all is said and done on this score, the fact remains that these forces are *outside* of us and even though they have an influence on us (which influence is the result of our own past actions), we have no control over them whatsoever! From the purely physical point of view, if it happens to be a difficult situation, the only choice we have is to be inactive and endure until this phase of planetary aspect changes. Then we can act and breathe again.

As long as an individual has not found his own center and Sun of Reality within, around which his life revolves, he is necessarily dependent on these outer forces to move him along like a leaf blown in the wind. We live either by an inner faith or are guided by outer circumstances. Which is our path and on what do we depend as our guiding star?

The forces outside are as impartial as the wind which blows. They affect us by the same vibratory energy waves which are latent within us and to which we respond. There are definite centers within us which correspond to certain centers in the universe. Like the air we breathe, radionic action of finer energies in the universe sustains our physical body. We have a definite relationship to these forces, but no control over them externally.

The amount of air taken into our body is governed by the act of breathing and the absorption of the oxygen and the energy in it. The finer energy circuits are also governed by centers and fields in our body which can be conditioned and positioned for energy flow from *our centers within*, when the without is not favorable. Primitive man had to endure the hardships of Nature, such as cold, heat, etc., as he had no means of complete isolation from without and very little means of duplicating these forces by reliable heat, ventilation, etc. In this age, that problem has been solved, but the other remains and leaves us as much a victim to outer forces in the finer energy fields as the cave man was to Nature's forces outside.

Man is a unit with a central sun and energy fields within himself in exact duplicate of the without, or he could not communicate and draw on the universal supplies needed to sustain the life in this body. Food, clothing and shelter are material things; but it is really the finer energies within these material things which we need the most!

The grossest must be expelled, as they act merely as conveyors and resistant substances of bulk to the process of life. The grosser material substances of too highly concentrated foods are often the cause of clogging the finer energy flow and circuits in the body. As a material agent, they act as effectively as unfavorable energy radiations from without, or as insufficient life radiations from the sun. Then the central core energy of the *individual life and sun* must be called upon to act, by polarizing its fields of body parts—which are positive, negative and neuter—in each field of the four modes of polarized motion in matter, like recharging a battery. The airy principle of life is involved here as the most important factor of oxidation, depending on elimination of the gross substances and their gases so the life process of oxidation can operate.

As the planets are positioned outside by rotation in their orbits, so man can take body postures which place the polarity energy fields—one immediately above the other—into action under a mild stress (or stretch) which forces them to work in two ways: first, by the electromagnetic polarity; second, by physical effort and gravity function, blended with the proper mental attitude. The body, the mind, and the subtle energies are therefore all engaged simultaneously.

Such are the fundamental postures illustrated in this book. In these postures, the calves of the legs are stretched and acted upon because they are the two most negative poles of the airy triad. The colon—the neuter pole of the airy fields—is acted upon by the posture and the pressure of the thighs upon it, plus the breath to activate the grosser substances of solids, liquids and gases, causing them to be expelled downward according to the law of Nature. Each field is placed as close as possible above the other, in active function. The chest and lungs form the positive pole and field of the airy principle. They are acted upon in the posture by the stretch of the back and the freeing of the brachial plexus for better action under that stimulus. Sound vibration with the breath adds to the stimulation of the central core. *Humming in high and low pitch can be used selectively to vibrate any area of the head or body where the hands are placed for polarization.*

The stretch through the breath—from within, outward—is also used several times in the posture shown in figure No. 3. The colon and the abdomen are well supported in this posture. In this way there is no danger of too much stress or strain on the abdominal walls, or for persons who may have a slight rupture. *Posture support is very important* until the muscles can be built up slowly by these simple, well-supported, muscle-stretch postures.

17

The House We Live In & Its Function

> "If we could only stand aside and see this grand Cinema of life in its Reality, we would become a most absorbed observer, in astonishment over the wonders that have been created for our use. We would then become the *witness* and the *viewer* instead of the idea that we are the *doer*. If we could do this, our 'toil would cease, our yoke would be easy and our burden light.' Then faith and love would rule."

The greatest mystery in the universe is man himself. Many forces and energies are at work in the body. Both wireless and conducted circuits (via nerves and tubes) carry on the wonderful work of the Creator in the human body. The human form is truly wonderfully made and maintained. The problem of how to keep it fit and useful for the longest period of service is an interesting one.

Our body is like the house we live in; when the electric currents are on, then light and heat are available. When the water pipes are in good shape and water is pumped through them by pressure, then all the fluid requirements are solved. When the gas is turned on, then cooking and gas heating are possible. And when the drainage is not obstructed, then the sewers do not back up and no regurgitation of drainage is pocketed in any part of the basement.

These are the functioning parts of our house, within its structure. A well built and well kept house will stand much strain and wear from daily use as well as from the elements. Such a house can be a very comfortable home for the persons living in it if they run and maintain it wisely. If something goes wrong in the function of it, or in the structure, is it the fault of the house or the dwellers in it who built it?

This is a startling thought when applied to our body. Certainly, when the house is neglected or the management of its mechanism is not understood, then it will not fulfill the requirements nor provide the comforts that are possible under wiser management. *The house does not condition the tenant in it, unless the dweller in it neglects the house.* Then any one of its automatic services can go wrong and the tenant can be very uncomfortable in the best constructed home.

The analogy of this house to our body (which we often think is the self) is a precise picture of the life of the soul, which is the *real* self, in the body. This *dweller* in the body is the Real Self. It functions through energies emanating from its being, as stepped-down currents of wireless circuits in its primary aspect. Mind is the first expression of the soul in matter. Mind is the finest essence of matter—as its neuter principle—around which positive and negative forces whirl and spin.

Matter has five phases, or fields of appearances. If the soul is to have experience in all matter, it must have it in all of its five phases: solids, liquids, gases, caloric energy as warmth and heat, and the etheric neuter as the medium of sensation.* (This latter includes the gustiferous ether conveying the electronic particles of taste, the luminiferous ether for sight, and so on through the five senses, working in five fields of etheric matter as sensory and motor functions.)

So, the mind is the first step-down of the soul's energy, as a neuter pole which expresses itself perfectly through the five sensory currents as five negative circuits and through the five motor currents as five positive expressions in all five fields of matter. These energies are originally wireless in their action as

---

*These five phases are referred to in many cultures and systems as the five elements, most commonly called earth, water, air, fire, and ether.

finer energy, or they could not contact the outside wireless fields of atomic construction and convey them inward, to the center, through further stepped-down and conducted currents over nerves and through tubes in the body. In this way, the consciousness within contacts and benefits by the energy fields in the macrocosmic world outside.

Mind, being a neuter activity in itself, is therefore capable of every capacity of action and sensation through matter. When properly controlled, it is a perfect servant of the soul, as a stepped-down expression of energy—both sensory and motor currents for the soul's experience in this world. The senses in turn are the five modes of expression of the mind in matter.

The luminiferous ether in the outer world is the conductor of light. Seeing is the function of the eyes in this ether, gathering rays from external objects through the lenses and reflecting them through the optic nerves, to the center of sight in the cuneus of the occipital lobe. The soniferous ether acts as a medium of sound conduction. The odoriferous ether acts as a conductor of fine gaseous particles for the perception of smell. The tactile ether acts as a conductor for the sense of touch. These wireless long-range contacts then travel over specific, conducted sensory receivers which carry the current inward to our inner sense-perception centers and are then registered as awareness or conscious experiences.

The mind expresses itself through its five stepped-down agencies—which split into the five sensory senses and the five motor senses—to carry on the work in the body as organic functions. These express themselves also as the mechanical leverages of ten fingers, for motion and expression of skill in overcoming gravity, and as ten toes and energy waves flowing to them for body motion through joints and leverage, conquering the inertia of their own matter in a world of gravity and resistance. These waves of energy give the delicate sense of touch to the fingers and create definite pattern lines of fingerprints in the tactile tissues. These are precise and unique in each individual, as is his brain pattern of perception waves in this life. The varieties are infinite, it seems, since no two finger-prints are exactly alike or they could not be used for identi-fication purposes.

Such delicate patterns and finer energy waves link our mental pattern to the outside world, to experience sensations through contact with matter in its five modes of resistance: through solid matter called *earth*, liquid matter called *water*, gaseous matter called *air*, heat or warmth called *fire*, and the etheric conductor of sensation for all four polarized elements —as the four sensory rivers of life out of our center of con-scious being, the Paradise within. When we see such definite functions of polarity through specific centers and body areas, we wonder if there is not a way to use these forces for better health and well-being.

The vital force of our being is located in the pelvic area, as the water principle. It has the eternal aspect of the seed power in itself, by which it can be used to create outside for *genera-tion* or by drawing on that force for body rebuilding, it can be used for *regeneration* of cells and structures inside. As a motor force, it is asleep in the space of the sacrum and has been spoken of as the "Kundalini" force, coiled like a serpent. Latent within the physical aspect of it are many mysteries of man's being.* The pelvis is the water-basin or reservoir of life's vital fluids. Instead of scattering or dissipating these currents, why not put them to their intended use through the posture stretches, thus utilizing this energy for regeneration, better health and general well-being?

This thought also is a startling discovery for those who will not admit a wireless anatomy or physiology function of our physical body but who credit the smallest particle of matter, the atom itself, with that very potent function. Is the body of

---

*See Dr. Stone's book *The Mysterious Sacrum* (included in Volume II of his Complete Collected Works) for more details on this energy and its mysteries.

man, as a composite, less than the smallest unit of its inherent matter? In our haste for weapons, which led to this discovery, have we forgotten the well-being of humanity, individually and as a whole? Having presented just sufficient groundwork to establish a reasonable basis for the wireless energy currents we intend to work with, we may proceed with the principles involved in the practice of this new idea of exercise that I've called Easy Stretching Postures.

It is through the efficiency of the wireless energy waves that this work is accomplished. This energy exists in the universe as a natural reservoir, and its energy circuits continue their course in man's body, over the brain tissue and the nerves of conduction. This finer energy also flows through the circulation as the life in the air, and through its electromagnetic action, it accomplishes the seemingly impossible feat of traveling through many miles of the finest capillary tubes, arteries, veins and lymph vessels. Without these finer energies, the mind could not operate the senses and benefit through experience in the wireless fields of the universe. This simple statement is almost as stupendous as Harvey's discovery of the circulation of the blood and may shape the healing art of the future.

The Easy Stretching Postures are based upon the function of this finer energy circulating in man's body and in the universe. Simplicity itself is the keynote. The basic squatting posture is as old as the race and as new as a child. Most little children automatically and unconsciously assume this posture while at play. Yet is must be rediscovered and personally tried by the individual—usually in the hour of need—in order to realize its value in enhancing energy current flow, which regulates his well-being.

A Posture for Better
Circulation of Energy Currents

When we mention exercise, we think only of muscular exertion, which taxes the body in order to promote better circulation. When the mind is occupied in a vigorous game, this effort is not so obvious, but just as strenuous and taxing for the poor heart muscle. With the advancing years in a man's life and the predominance of heart ailments everywhere, few physicians will take the chance of recommending strenuous exercise after the age of fifty, or even before, according to the health of the patient.

Then what is the poor man or woman going to do with all the tension that is still in the mind and in the emotions, and with all the gas in the uncomfortable abdomen? And who is not bothered with excess gas in these days of hurrying and injudicious selection of quantity, quality and combinations of food? Is walking for miles the only possible answer for emotional tension? Is it practical for most patients?

What has this new finding to offer for this common condition, as well as for many minor ailments which gradually develop into serious conditions of ill health? What simple thing can one do to preserve bodily functions at par and stay well, or even to regain health with the expenditure of the least amount of effort and time? The answer is an Easy Stretching Posture which is so natural that it takes only three to five minutes, once or several times a day if necessary, to increase the release of gases and the consequent intake and absorption of oxygen in the body, and to quickly release mental and emotional tension.

18

The Airy Principle as a Triune Function in the Body

"Never force anything, physically or mentally!"

Life begins with breath. With a cry the babe enters this world, and the aged leave it with a sigh. The airy principle in Nature is the most important in life's function. Not even one cell can live without air, much less function without it.

The air is a neuter principle in Nature and links man's respiratory life essence with its own by constant exchange of inhalations and exhalations—centripetal and centrifugal action —a positive and a negative flow. And on what does this exchange depend? On the positive factor of forceful breathing? Not nearly as much as we think! The elimination of the negative factor of carbon dioxide in the blood and tissues, as well as other waste gases, is the final answer to this circuit of inhalation and expulsion of all gases which clog and block the cells of the body. *Oxygen cannot be taken up by the blood in the presence of carbon dioxide or other waste gases in the blood.* The presence of one real gas bubble in the circulation can be serious; and diffused gases will not permit oxidation in the tissues, except in the lungs which have a special arrangement for the escape of carbon dioxide gases through the very thin membranes of the lung tissues.

Stagnant waste gases are often absorbed by the thin layers of the endoderm, or lining in the bowels, especially in the colon, because in the arrangement of fields in the body, the colon is the neuter pole for the airy principle, where the gases accumulate like in a reservoir. The lungs act as a positive pole or intake, and superior pole exchange of exhaust through exhalation. For perfect health and vitality, these energy fields must co-ordinate as positive, neuter and negative functions of life and elimination.

When the neuter reservoir is loaded with gases and the exit is not functioning properly, the back pressure goes through the tissues of the body as shooting pains anywhere, also producing spasms of the diaphragm known as hiccoughs. In such a condition, pressure on nerve reflex areas in the abdomen will cause head symptoms to appear via the pneumogastric nerve current reflex as well as the diffused gases in the blood stream and tissues. Indigestion and the resulting gaseous end products of fermentation are responsible for excess gases in the colon, which is their natural place of storage.

Indigestion is one of the most common complaints of young and old. Babies cry because of it, youngsters bend over with their hands pressing on the abdomen, and old folks moan when the gas pressure and its resulting pain is too severe.

The normal temperature in the stomach is 105 degrees F. and about 106 F. in the small intestines. Gastric juices are secreted by the mucous membranes of the stomach and pour over the food as it is mixed and churned in the stomach. When enough of this fluid is secreted, it preserves the food during the process of digestion. However, if this fiery energy is diverted to other parts at this time, then the digestion is incomplete and the food sours and ferments, belching being a natural evidence of this condition.

The amount of food put into the stomach at one time, the quality, the combination, and at what temperature, are all important factors in the process of digestion, assimilation in the small intestines, and elimination through the colon. The colon is the gathering place and the natural storage area of waste and gases. Any solid matter or gas which has passed through the iliocecal valve must be eliminated downward.

The natural exit for all colonic gases is the anus. Even though the outlet is so near the reservoir, it is often very difficult to expel the gases. There are many mechanical answers in books, but they help little when one has a real belly-ache due to gas pains. The squatting postures assist this process as well as the general currents of energy flowing downward for the digestive and eliminative processes.

Gas pains are one of the main post-operative problems, for which the good doctor has no pills. Even allowing the patient to move around soon after an operation, while it helps, is not the answer to the problem. Then what is? The answer is that there is a downward function of energy in Nature, called "apana" in the Eastern terms of old, which is embodied in the airy principle and causes the normal expulsion or elimination in the lower, natural outlets of the body—*and this is activated by the squatting posture* and by Polarity Therapy. Even in childbirth, this is the active principle which causes the delivery of the baby. It is the current which flows over these abdominal and pelvic muscles and causes them to contract. The primitive tribes had this ancient knowledge as a heritage from their ancestors, and women would take a natural, squatting posture for delivery. In their natural state of good health, childbirth seldom delayed the moving tribes.

It would be helpful to expectant mothers to prepare and condition the pelvis for the delivery of the child. The muscles of the pelvic floor could be toned and made more elastic by these simple stretching postures, beginning immediately after conception. In the later stages of pregnancy, let the physician in charge decide what is best. If one has cultivated the habit of taking these postures long before conception and in the early stages of pregnancy, it may also relieve or eliminate the excruciating leg pains with which pregnant women are often troubled. Even after childbirth, the easy stretching postures help in restoring the normal figure.

Pains in the calves of the legs: When these pains are not due to circulatory obstructions in the veins and arteries as a result of long endured stagnant pressure in the current flow, *then they are reflex gas pains from the colon downward,* as the neuter airy pole acting on the negative pole in the calves of the legs. The colon has a specific reflex area in the calf of each leg, between the fibula and tibia, as is explained and shown in Charts 60 and 61 in the Supplement to *The Wireless Anatomy of Man.** When this most negative area of the airy triad is stimulated, release is obtained by reflex polarity of the fields of air in the body. It is not a nerve reflex of physiology, as far as nerve tracing has shown. *It works by a prior positioning of polar opposites in the elements of matter in their grouping of principles in action on polarity fields.*

The reason for giving this lengthy description of the principles involved is to enable the reader to understand the real problem which is not usually covered in books on similar subjects. Without understanding the principle, the practice does not succeed nor endure. These postures are so simple that one cannot value them or persevere in their practice unless *one knows what he is doing and why.* The results will speak for themselves. The postures are not so easy to take as they look. We are more bound and stiff than we realize!

The energy current of the internal downward force must be activated by stimulating all three areas of the airy field at once, so the exit and the inlet—the negative pole first, then the positive one—can function with precision as designed by the Creator. The squatting posture is the most natural position to favor the current of expulsion from above, downward. The posture is so simple and obvious that we may choose to pass it by and continue to suffer.

After years of study of every health posture and exercise, including the eighty-four Yoga postures, I have found none equal to this one which combines squatting and stretching for

---

*See Volume I of Dr. Stone's Complete Collected Works.

relaxation and well-being. It gives the most results for the thing which nearly everybody needs—freeing of gases and supplying more air and oxidation for the body. For the minimum of time and effort spent for health, none can equal it in results. It has even deeper values for higher benefits not touched upon here. A few minutes spent each day for relief of gases and improved elasticity of muscles will be rewarded by better energy flow.

With the downward current active as the most negative function, namely elimination, all other functions are free to act without that drag of all the waste products of solids, liquids and gases in the tissues of the body. When even one bubble of air in a hot water or steam pipe can cause the whole system to pound like hammers and stop all circulation in an inanimate object, what must it be in a living organism! When the principle involved is once understood, the Easy Stretching Postures will come naturally as they are tried. Anyone may be convinced by the benefits derived from the exercises. But, in the beginning, it should be practiced for only two or three minutes at a time, *without forcing anything.*

Some may think that merely squatting when defecating is sufficient. But that is not enough. I have tried this posture for years in that manner without much gain or awakening of its importance as the quickest road to health and elasticity of muscles and balance of motion, until the posture was taken as an exercise and combined with the stretches illustrated in this book.

This springy step is possible by gentle perseverance only. Do not force! *Nature's way is gentle growth.* Gradual change marks her path everywhere. *When Nature moves suddenly, it is for destruction.* No wonder the ancients likened Nature's forces to angry gods who strike swiftly and powerfully!

19
Digestion & the Fiery Energy

"Life must flow, or it leaves the form, or body, and the shell is dead when the life is not in it. Love is the gateway of life. . . . Where there is love, there is life. Love is not a duty; it is life itself. When the personal emotions crowd out the true Love energy and essence of Life, then there are created blocks of interference which cause great suffering—physically, mentally and emotionally. Such a one punishes himself by mental and emotional fixation and selfish determination. The soul starves for lack of the water of Love, of Forgiveness, of the real vision and purpose of life.

"Many physical pains, rheumatic and arthritic fixations in joints are due to a stoppage of this Life Energy flow because of mental or emotional dams in the conscious or subconscious field of mind energy. That is why hatred, jealousy, pride and even entertaining grief are considered sins against the Holy Ghost, the Spirit of Life within us. All these blocks, self-created and maintained as fixations, 'are not forgiven', said Jesus briefly.

"Only the floodgates of a greater Love can be the answer to these personal grievances and fixations. Forgiveness is a natural process in a life full of Love. It is natural to the Saints, to the Sages, the Mystics and little children. No wonder Jesus said that we must become as little children in order to enter the kingdom of heaven. Heaven is where love flows freely and impersonally. It is the Oneness of life and it is the One Real Essence."

At last we come to the problem of digestion, which is much improved by using the squatting posture because it releases natural energy currents plus the gases and end products of elimination. For years I noticed that illness usually starts in the digestive region, because the downward expelling force is not working. We call it constipation, but it is much more than that. The bulk of the retained feces causes less trouble than we think. It is the gases and the inactive airy force that actually back up to the positive pole, like the sewer gas which kills more often than the backwash of sewage. It doesn't all arise from the backwash, but from the total in the pipes. We are prone to put too much emphasis on the material solid evidence and too little on the *blocked energy field* and *blocked current flow* which is the *real cause* of the physical stagnation.

Energy, when turned on, can move any amount of bulk. But mere bulk can move nothing. And still the quantity impresses us more than the quality of the evidence! Our experience with atomic forces will change all our material viewpoints in time. If we want to be in the advance guard of progress, there is no time like NOW! As we sow, so we reap.

It will be helpful to understand a little more about our digestion, as faulty digestion is responsible for the excess gases and much ill health. *Digestion is a fire which consumes material.* In the mythologies of the Norsemen, the earth was considered a huge body, and in the abdomen, or in the bowels of the earth, lived the god Vulcan, who was a fire God. He had a smithy and a forge in that hot place in the middle of the earth, where he forged the chains for those condemned by the gods. It is an interesting story when we consider the import of what these myths are trying to tell us in the form of symbols and stories. Can we read what is written therein for our benefit? Man forges many chains of ills with his own knife and fork at the dining table; and how compelling are the bonds of sickness.

"Those whom the gods condemned" implies those who disregard the wisdom of the laws of life, the purpose higher than mere indulgence of the appetites and the senses. Those lacking in intelligent self-control become victims of indulgence and are bound by their own limitations, created in the depths of their own nature. Energies become bonds when stagnant, blocked, or when reversed through our own improper use or abuse. Such is the story our Norse ancestors left in their archives for the benefit of those who wish to profit thereby.

Digestion as a Fire in a Boiler

This is a simple and practical illustration that can do much to carry home just one point. Food must be digested just as fuel must be burnt, or clinkers remain. If the good reader ever fired a furnace or a boiler in a power plant, he learned a few very valuable lessons, namely:

1st — Not too much shoveled in at once.

2nd — Spread the coal *thinly* over the hot embers.

3rd — Regulate the draft.

4th — Select the fuel which will burn best—leaving the least amount of clinkers—with the least fumes and smoke.

If persons are sincere in their effort to gain or regain health, these four points are invaluable as guides to the principles of combustion, inside or outside the body. No one wants to be preached to all the time about diet, etc. We ourselves must do a little observing and selecting as to quantity, combinations and quality of foods taken at each meal. It becomes an interesting study when we have a purpose in mind, like firing a locomotive to run better and pull more freight. We all want service from our bodies and from our automobiles. Do we care as much for our own body, which does the actual important work, as we do for the car which merely takes us there?

Our actual needs for food and fuel are so simple and so few, but they must be in keeping with our mind and our desires, or else we feel frustrated. If we continue to observe the reactions from our own eating habits, we will soon learn, like the little boy who ate green apples. Nature teaches and we can easily learn by being apt pupils; but if indulgence is our aim, then suffering is the result—sooner or later. Why should we pay such a high price for that little pleasure of eating? Simple foods serve best, and they should be neither too rich, nor fried, nor too sweet. Simplicity in diet helps much in the process of digestion. Less combinations at any one meal makes the work easier for the stomach. Another very important factor is a cheerful attitude, especially at meal time. It is better not to eat at all when one is upset. At a time like that, it is best to limit the intake to hot liquids.

Be your own engineer and study the fires of your body and what results you get from them in fuel consumption. We observe this in our house's boiler or furnace, and the gasoline mileage in our car; is the body less important to us?

We either constrain ourselves and intelligently govern our appetites, or Nature does it for us; but then we don't learn why constraint was necessary and we suffer ill health besides.

20

The Health Postures & Their Stages of Accomplishment

"You don't have to go to extremes in the postures. . . . Skill just requires greater concentration."

The basic posture stretch should be done in the middle of a room on a soft rug, with nothing behind the person, so that if the balance is lost, it will be just an easy roll on a rug—like a rocking motion—as the buttocks are only a few inches from the floor in these postures. It does not take a large space at all, just enough so one does not bump against anything if the balance is lost while attempting to take the position, which happens frequently until one gets used to the squatting posture. The balance is easily maintained forward and sideways, and no extra space is needed in these two directions; it is only the space in back of the person which should be clear for a roll.

The feet should be *flat* on the floor for the muscle stretch on the legs. Merely placing the weight on the balls of the feet or on the toes does not give the best results. It is better to try to do a little stretching right then and there than to place the weight on the balls of the feet or toes in this posture. If necessary, it can be done with shoes on at first, since the heels are a lift and less stretching of the muscles of the calves are required if the heels are slightly elevated. The same heel lift for this posture may be accomplished by using a small pad under the heels. However, for the maximum benefit, it is best

128

done barefooted and without support under the heels, after one gets accustomed to the posture.

Clothing should be loose and free in order to get the most value out of the few minutes spent in this stretching posture. Pajamas or shorts are ideal for it. If done in other clothing, like trousers or slacks, gently test their range of giving in the direction you are going—or they will part company! Also, the range of stretch that can be accomplished will be far too limited in tight clothing.

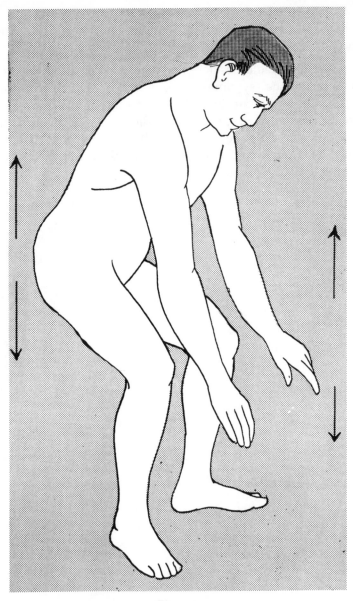

Fig. I

PREPARATORY POSITION WITH UP AND DOWN ROCKING MOTION TO
GET INTO THE SQUATTING POSTURE

Figure 1 shows the preliminary stage of gently rocking—while moving downward—a little at a time, until the posture shown in figure 2 is attained, or as far as one can comfortably get down, without strain or force.

The arrows indicate the up-and-down rocking motion for achieving the squatting position.

The feet should be about six inches apart at the heels and about twelve inches apart at the toes. This will differ a little with each person as his comfort or balance permits.

The close position of the feet gives more support to the abdomen by the thighs pressing on nearly all of it from the anterior, especially when the knees are pushed together as shown in figure 3, for expelling gas and stimulating the downward currents which govern the peristaltic movement of the bowels.

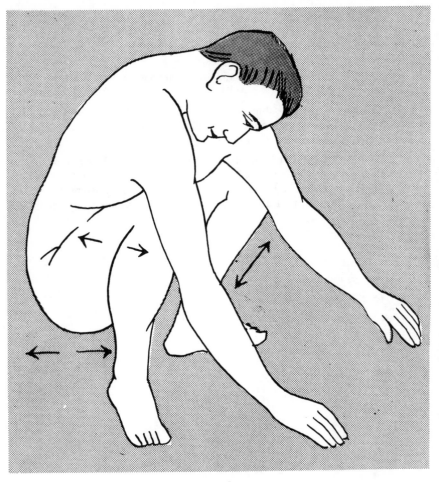

Fig. 2

HEALTH POSTURE COMPLETED WITH THE ARMPITS RIGHT OVER THE KNEES,
ROCKING IN ALL DIRECTIONS FOR RELEASE

Figure 2 shows the completion of the squat, with the armpits right over the knees. The thighs support the abdomen. The feet are flat on the floor *and stay there*. Now the rocking motion is started from the anterior to the posterior—forward and backward—then laterally, from one side to the other; and also rotating around the center pivot of the spine. The latter is like the side movement, but it adds a twisting stretch to the muscles of the pelvis.

These gentle efforts of rocking make one forget the posture, by taking the stress and strain away from one set of muscles and throwing them on the opposite group, like a teeter-totter. This is very useful in accomplishing the posture and for resting the muscles alternately. It also has a stimulating effect through polarity function, from the positive to the negative side, around an imaginary neuter line of gravity, through the center of the spine.

The hands are stretched out, *but do not touch the floor*. This is merely for assurance until the posture becomes steady and natural while the rocking is done.

Great relaxation is attained, as the armpits rest right on the knees; it also adds the polarity action of the fields to its value.

The posture, including the rocking, can all be done in one minute, once it has been mastered.

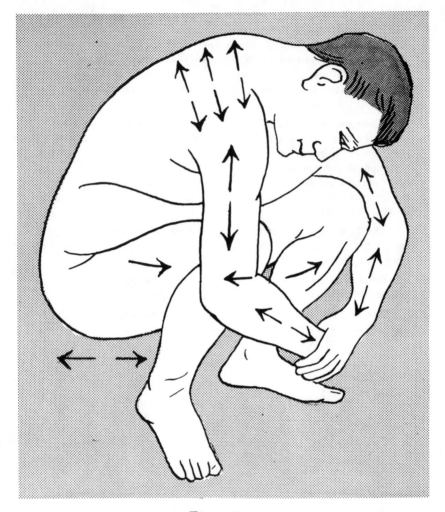

Fig. 3

HEALTH POSTURE COMPLETE WITH STRETCHES ON ARMS, KNEES
AND SPINE, FOR GAS RELEASE AND CONSTIPATION.

Figure 3 is the same as figure 2 except that the arms are *wrapped around the knees from the outside,* and the knees are pushed together to stretch an entirely new set of muscles while rocking back and forth, from side to side, and also in a rotating motion.

The push inward, toward the middle, exerted on both knees, acts like a fulcrum for the arm stretch and is felt in the hip joints, freeing them from blocks and tension, for easier walking with a spring in the step, and makes the body feel light due to releasing muscles locked in the daily gravity-pull position. The amount of the push is regulated by each person according to tolerance and comfort. *NO FORCE IS USED.* It is only a gentle persuasion through a rocking motion which does it, little by little, like a seesaw. *Playful exertion* is the general idea. Poise and general well-being are accomplished without compulsion, by rhythmic movements in relaxed positions.

Next, the locked hands exert a stretch upon the arms and between the shoulders, to free the brachial plexus. The head is bent forward and the spine is extended in this process. *The pull must be felt between the shoulders to be effective.* A deep breath is taken, stretching from the inside out, to relax tension and energy blocks. This is a lift and extension on the cavity walls from within to counteract the outer pressure and tension from daily work that is placed on external muscles and the structures of the body. The breath is directed to act as a push from within, between the shoulders, while the arms pull on the shoulders from without, in a synchronized stretch. A healthy grunt as the breath is exhaled helps deep relaxation.

Not only is the spine extended in this process, but sometimes even vertebrae will reposition themselves with a gentle click. It is a lift upward from within, by the breath, without force or strain. This is a purely physical stretch. The breath is directed to one area at a time and synchronized with the muscle-stretch on that place outside. No effort is made at any other kind of breath control or regulation. Daily efforts are necessary to follow through with the currents so liberated.

After a satisfactory stretch, the breath is released with a grunt, which adds to the relaxation. Even sick persons can groan themselves into well-being, if the principle is understood and if the effort is deep enough to arouse the latent life forces dormant in the body. Many animals do this instinctively when they roll on the ground and grunt most satisfactorily after a hard day's work in the harness. A great English physician once said: "The gallant Frenchman will groan himself well while the stolid Englishman succumbs to the malady." Such observations of man's deeper reserve forces put to good use *by action* have been made by many other doctors, especially in time of crisis and severe illness.

The arrows on the arms and shoulder indicate the pull which is exerted by the locked hands, *with arm leverage around the knees,* stretching the muscles between the shoulder blades and freeing the brachial plexus. A circuit of energy flow is established from the locked hands to the back.

This posture is ideal for the release of gases, constipation, excessive abdominal fat, and for toning the walls of the abdomen by the muscular exertion and squeezing by the thighs, which also protects the muscles from excess strain in this posture.

This stretching exercise activates fields and muscle tissues which rarely get any exercise in the entire day's work. Joints will become free, walking will be easier, the step more elastic, and there will be less heaviness due to stagnation and gases in the abdomen because the posture eliminates this sluggishness. Even the cheeks will glow, and the heart and lungs can benefit greatly by this stretch of the brachial area.

The real currents at work are the life currents in the airy principle, with their upward and downward action behind every inspiration and exhalation of air. One minute or so is sufficient to start the currents.

21

Youth Posture for Balance & Elasticity

"When you realize that you do nothing, you don't get tired."

Vital force resides latent in the pelvis; anteriorly, it is the generative and regenerative force; and posteriorly, it is the latent motor force, sometimes called the "Kundalini", asleep in the spinal fluids of the sacral area—as a motor force within the three-walled enclosure of the dura mater, arachnoid and pia mater membranes. *This force can be utilized to activate and rebuild the body through concentrated effort of a few minutes of regular, daily, stretching postures.*

The brain is the positive motor pole for *mind action*, while the pelvis is the negative motor pole for *physical action*. The pelvis contains the latent force and drive behind all our actions, whether we are aware of it or not. It represents all the involuted mental and emotional energy which is concentrated here for physical exertion and expression. Even the arms could not swing freely nor act without the support of the fixed pelvis, by muscular co-ordination. It is the foundation of the deep, as the seed power energy field at the base of physical life. Situated anteriorly in the pelvis is the sensory current and a structural force for life-form building, while the motor force is in the posterior part of the pelvis. All the sensory currents— whether emanating from the brain or the pelvis—have their centers in the anterior part of the body, while all the motor currents have their centers in the posterior portion.

The Youth Posture shown in figure 4 starts a new series of stretches, effectively utilizing this latent energy in the pelvis

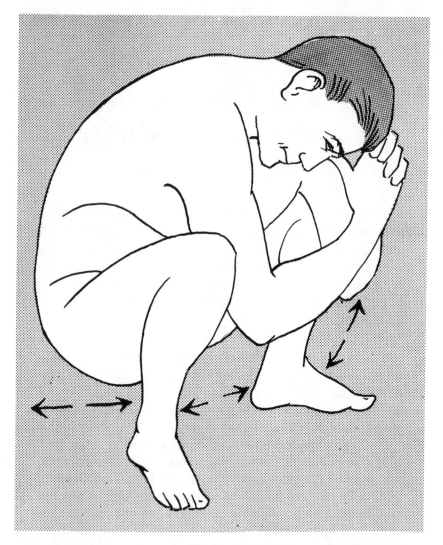

Fig. 4

YOUTH POSTURE WITH FEET FARTHER APART   FOR GREATER
STRETCH ON OPPOSITE GROUPS OF MUSCLES AND THE HIP JOINTS

when freed by posture stretches. Polarity currents are activated and distributed by the hands from the positive and negative sides of the body. The triune principle of polarity is used
throughout this work as finer energies and fields in action.

The exercise illustrated in figure 4 emphasizes muscular
elasticity, through the stimulation of the finer currents behind
their activity. Normal exchange of all currents and energy
waves through the tissues expresses itself as health, elastic
response and balance, and as relaxation.

For this posture, we rock into position as gently as for the
one shown in figure 1; but here *the feet are farther apart* to
begin with, for more stretch and muscular motion and the
freedom attained thereby. The heels should be twelve inches
or more apart, and the toes about twenty-four inches or so.
The exact distance will vary because muscles differ in tone
and elasticity. Accordingly, each one must find his measure
and start gently. So this should be done gradually by the individual, as it can be comfortably tolerated. Benefits are obtained with the least amount of effort.

It is not accomplishment of a position that we are after,
but *the stimulating actions of the currents set into motion by
these posture stretches.* Those who need them the most will
at first feel that they accomplished the least, but they will
slowly feel the benefits just the same. *It is like turning on a
switch and allowing the currents to do the work,* instead of
wasting a lot of energy in performing acrobatic stunts. All this
is based on Nature's finer forces in motion.

In this posture, the arms are placed on the *inside* of the
knees, *pushing the knees outward* in order to stretch the
inner and posterior groups of muscles. The palm and fingers
of one hand are placed over the loosely formed fist of the
other hand, placing the thumbs side by side—one on each side
of the bridge of the nose, in an upward direction—thus supporting the head with the thumbs, while both arms are resting
between the two knees, as shown in the illustration.

Having assumed the posture, we proceed with the rocking motions as before—forward, backward, side to side, and rotational. Here entirely new muscle groups come into play for unlocking stagnant forces within them and releasing active energy blocks. The currents thus liberated are used in the succeeding posture applications explained in the following chapters. The posture stretching exercises described so far constitute a complete series of daily exercise for general health maintenance. But for persons who need special help, a series of self-help applications have been added in Chapter 22 and are based on the same foundation: namely, allowing the released currents to do the work as Nature intended.

PLEASE NOTE: THE POSTURE STRETCHING EXERCISES CONTAINED IN THIS BOOK ARE INTENDED FOR THE MAINTENANCE OF NORMAL HEALTH AND, THROUGH BETTER ENERGY FLOW, THE IMPROVEMENT OF DRAGGING, SUB-NORMAL, CHRONIC CONDITIONS WHICH DO NOT READILY RESPOND TO THE USUAL REMEDIES AND TREATMENT. THE OBJECT OF THIS PRESENTATION IS *NOT SELF-DIAGNOSIS OR SELF-TREATMENT* IN CASE OF ILLNESS. WHEN ILL, *DO CONSULT YOUR PHYSICIAN.*

Youthfulness as Physical & Spiritual Health

In kidney trouble these squatting postures are also very helpful as a home remedy. The squatting exercise frees the space of pressure and gases where the kidneys are, and the downward airy energy of "apana" can then function more freely in expelling wastes—solids, liquids, or gases. When the body becomes water-logged and too heavy, it is because the kidneys are not functioning enough.

It has been observed that in all cases of chronic indigestion, the kidneys do not function freely. Their overnight output is very small in quantity, when the repair of tissue and drainage should be taking place. The process of digestion is also dependent on the downward flow of the life energy to accomplish the combustion and oxidation of foods and liquids.

If the elimination of the waste matter lags, then there is a back pressure which slows down the entire procedure and we call it indigestion. In this condition, the foods lay inactive in the stomach and ferment. The temperature there is normally 105° Fahrenheit. This warmth is needed for the digestion of foods, but it causes souring or fermentation of foods when they remain too long in the stomach and when they are not churned properly by the energy in the stomach and mixed with the natural hydrochloric acid secretions of the stomach walls, which are liberated in this churning and secretive action.

Again we find here that energy travels in *circuits* of Polarity Currents, *where the beginning and the end processes depend on each other.* It is a series of sequences rather than isolated factors. It seems as though *the first is last and the last is first* in the Polarity sequences of life's wheel.

In explaining these simple facts to mothers, they usually tell me that they have observed their younger children to take the squatting posture naturally before they go to potty. The posture usually precedes the function of elimination. However, it is done so naturally and regularly that it often escapes the attention of the parents. Since this instinctive procedure of adopting this posture for elimination is given as a heritage to babes, who do it unconsciously, could it indeed be valuable for grown-ups to use regularly when mastered once again, to regain a small fraction of the naturalness and youthfulness of childhood? Truly, it is said that Truth is revealed in its simplicity from the mouths of babes and sucklings.

Also, many of the postures and seemingly unimportant actions of children have a more direct relation to the Life within than we can fathom. Life in that stage expresses itself freely and spontaneously. When we see youth take these postures naturally and frequently during each day, could we call these postures by any other name than "The Easy Stretching Postures of Youth and Natural Beauty of Childhood"? There is a great cry for naturalness in this Iron Age of strain and tension. And again it is said, "A little child shall lead them." This can be literally applied. We all seek the freedom of the felicity of childhood and the naturalness of that way of Life. But we fail to adopt even one of the measures of exercise taken by the children of Life, whom we envy in their natural glee and radiance of Life's Energy Currents.

Happiness comes from within outward and rests in the love and security of the child in its dependence on its parents. As children of God, could not grown-ups have the same faith and love toward their Creator? The simplicity of Life as seen in children eliminates mental conditioning. Life has its own path and it is not that of the mind and its calculations. Faith, hope, love and humility are spiritual qualities and are not products of our mind but rather are a heritage of the soul, the great gifts of eternal verity from the all-beneficent Creator.

Possessions and toys are but occupations for the mind and its exercise, *which do not add one iota to the lasting happiness of children or grown-ups.* When a child is hungry or wants love, help or attention, it leaves all its toys and runs to mother or father. Could not all the grown-ups in this "Kindergarten of Life" adopt the same procedure of natural, soulful living, regardless of creeds? Is there any religion which does not advocate the practice of simple spiritual principles in daily life? Since health is a natural sequence of a balanced life, it cannot be neglected if we wish to be free and enjoy life to the fullest as real children of God.

There are a few things which *we ourselves must do daily to keep in tune with Life and its waves of radiance*, broadcasting from centers within our being and from the cosmos outside. If our mind energy and attention are too much occupied with toys and outer things which change daily, then we lose that fine touch with our inner Life and its loving care and radiance gained by "dwelling under the wings of the Almighty." Therefore, all grown-ups should consciously walk with God every hour and with every breath, *and all will be given unto them.* The mind becomes harsh and dominant *when we forget our Creator for even one moment.* We enjoy the gifts of life but, alas, we forget the Great Giver of all when success crowns our efforts. It is then that all sweetness and loveliness of life departs and the materially successful person becomes merely a caretaker of many "things".

When there was struggle and insecurity in the earlier days of life, when the children were young, there was happiness and a bond of love and unity in all. Now, there is material security which is depended upon, and that radiance of life passes that "Egyptian's door" whose first-born attention is not to God, the Creator of all and the Giver of all good. When man becomes so successful in the world that he does not need to thank God with every breath, *then indeed he stands alone.* Even the Savior of mankind passes by that heart's door because it is closed to love.

22

A Self-Help Series
of Postures for
Special Conditions

*"Ninety per cent of pain is emotional. Imag-
ination is our worst enemy. There is a spasm
in the emotional field before the spasm in
the spine and the body."*

The normalizing posture illustrated in figure 5 can be used
as a correction for flat dorsal spines. It is the same as the posture shown in figure 4 with the exception that the hands are
placed on the back of the head for a *mild stretch of the entire
spine*, from top to bottom. A gentle forward-and-backward
rocking motion is indicated by the arrows. A deep breath is
taken and used as a stretch from within, directed to any one
portion of the spine at one time, then released with a healthy
grunt.

The hands may be placed on any area from the neck to
the top of the head, to bring out a greater curve and stretch
on the spine wherever it is needed. *The pull must be very
gentle*, as we are working with great leverage here. A gentle
physical stretch, a stretch from within by the use of the
breath, and a rocking motion are the main factors in this
posture.

This posture stretch, for example, frees muscle tension
and energy blocks from the heart area, where anterior verte-
bral positions of the spine often interfere with its function.
Spinal checks have proved this to be the case in many in-
stances. A protruding chest often indicates an anterior curve

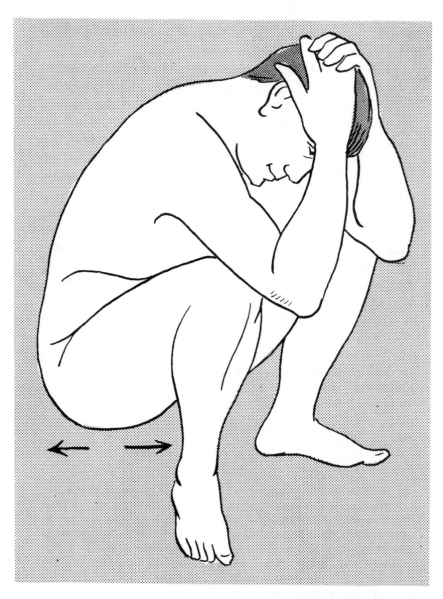

Fig. 5

THE YOUTH POSTURE WITH A SPINAL STRETCH.

and stress in the dorsal spine, which acts as a block to natural current flow and nerve transmission of energy.

This posture is also very beneficial to spines which lack the natural posterior dorsal curve. The higher on the back the flatness of the spine appears, the higher the hold on the head must be. In lower dorsal flatness of the spine, the hold is lower on the neck, in order to bring out the spine posteriorly in that area, until normal compensation remains in the musculature. One-half minute of this rocking stretch is sufficient *if repeated daily.*

After these exercises, when relaxation is complete, grasping a bar with both hands and hanging from it usually releases a number of vertebrae in a general spinal stretch. This stretch on the spine, arms and shoulders by hanging lifts the gravity compression from the articulating joints and from the cartilages between them, and it completes the stretch from above downward, as a gravity lift. This is also a fine stretch that compensates for the downward position of the hands in lifting objects and working all day long. It is easy to install a one-and-a-half inch curtain pole in any doorway. When it is so conveniently located, one is more apt to make good use of it by hanging from it as mentioned above, for a minute or so after having taken the posture stretching exercises, or at any time.

The position of the body for the stretching exercise shown in figure 6 is the same as shown in figure 5 but uses a contact with one hand placed on the back of the head and extending down over part of the neck, with the head bent to one side, for a stretch on the side of the spine and back that is troublesome, tense, or limited in motion. Either hand may be used and either side may be stretched, depending on where it is needed. This exercise also frees the brachial plexus on that side where the pull is felt. It is done *gently, only once or twice each time,* but regularly when it is needed. On the left, the pull can be felt over the posterior heart region, and on the right side it is felt over the liver region, acting as a release there.

When there is pain between the shoulders, any or all of these applications can be used with great benefit. Each posture approaches the condition from a different angle. We start with a current release and end in a muscular stretch. The field of finer forces and the overall current flow are our first considerations, and then the specific and local applications of polarity in all its phases and fields, including the outer forces of leverage and gravity.

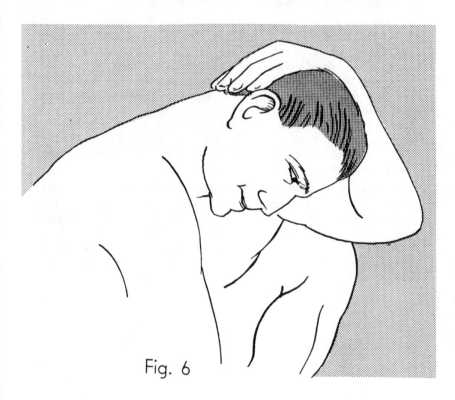

Fig. 6

YOUTH POSTURE WITH A STRETCH ON ONE SIDE OF THE NECK WHERE TENSION EXISTS.

The postures shown in figures 7 and 8 are the same as in figures 4 and 5 except that in 7 and 8 both hands are used for the eyes. Two illustrations are given to show the exact position of the hands and fingers, as this is very important for polarity reactions. The hands fit naturally over the sides of the face: the thumbs behind the jaw, directly under the ears; and the lower palms supporting the angle of the lower jaw; the other three fingers on the side of the head.

The little finger of each hand is the actor here. It pushes gently ON THE EYEBALLS, RIGHT UP UNDER THE ORBITAL RIDGE, to free the eyeball from its tension and soreness. The contact is gently applied for a few seconds *wherever soreness and tension may be found, until the whole area over the eyeball has been taken care of.* Each sore spot is held for a few seconds or up to one minute, to release the energy blocks. The gentle push upward regulates the pressure used. A very highpitched humming sound is made by using the breath from within until that area seems to respond to it by feeling the vibrations in it. This is done for about one minute or more daily, if there is need of it. Surprising results may be noted. Be sure the nails on the little fingers are cut short!

The center of sight is in the cuneus of the occipital lobe. In eye strain or eye trouble, blocks are present in the center which register as soreness about the middle of the occipital bone, behind the ear, on each side of the back of the head. Contact made there, accompanied by a humming sound, with the thumb on the sore spots on each side, placing the supporting fingers over the forehead, can polarize this area and relieve the soreness by repeated efforts.

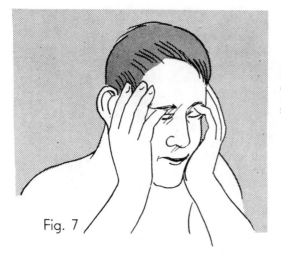

YOUTH POSTURE FOR EYE EXER-
CISE WITH THE LITTLE FINGER
PUSHING UP GENTLY UNDER THE
SUPRA ORBITAL RIM, TO FREE EN-
ERGY BLOCKS AND TENSION

Fig. 7

SIDE VIEW OF THE POSITION
OF THE HANDS

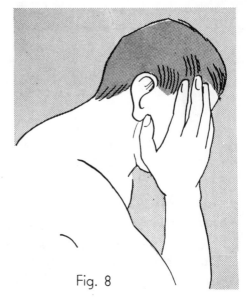

Fig. 8

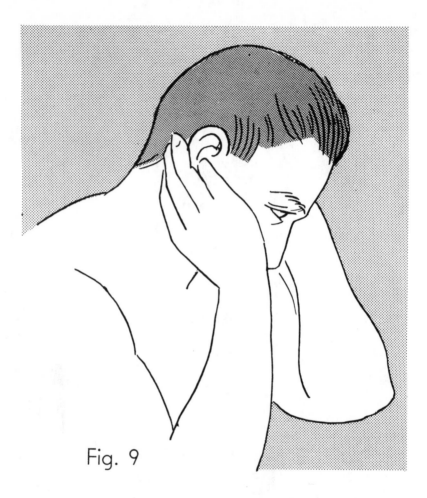

Fig. 9

YOUTH POSTURE FOR ENERGY RELEASE IN THE EARS BY
PLACING THE LITTLE FINGER OF EACH HAND IN EACH EAR,
PLUS HUMMING THE PROPER PITCH TO VIBRATE THE EAR
CANAL

Figure 9 illustrates self-help by means of the current of sound for balance and elasticity, for general central reaction in the middle area of the head, for ear trouble, head noises, etc. The position of the body is the same as that shown in figure 5.

The little finger of each hand is placed in each ear, giving the canal a lifting motion as well as dilating it. The lower jaw may be opened and shut a few times to augment the reaction at the joints. Now hold the little fingers still, keeping them inserted as far as comfortable into the ear canal, and hum different pitches of sound until you hear and feel the vibrations in the ear, just where the trouble is. Keep this up for one minute. If the trouble is more on one side than the other, then leave the finger in that ear only and withdraw the other one.

For a condition in the middle ears, press equally with both fingers and hum, and the sound will be about in the center of the head. Vary the pitch and the application to your needs. Much can be done by daily practice.

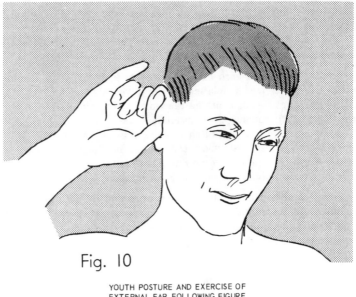

Fig. 10

YOUTH POSTURE AND EXERCISE OF
EXTERNAL EAR, FOLLOWING FIGURE
NINE WITH HUMMING FOR VIBRATION
BY SOUND IMPACT

The same posture as shown in figure 5 is held while using the normalizing ear exercise shown in figure 10. Insert the thumb in one ear and grasp that ear lobe with the first finger, then pull and rotate gently, humming all the time the right pitch for this outer part to respond and vibrate.

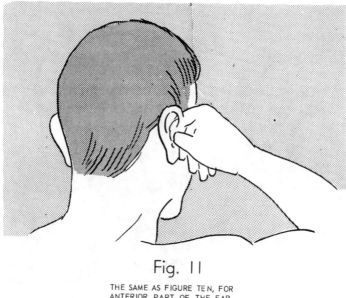

Fig. 11

THE SAME AS FIGURE TEN, FOR
ANTERIOR PART OF THE EAR,
CALLED THE TRAGUS

For the exercise shown in figure 11 we maintain the same squatting position which liberates the general overall currents, while continuing the ear exercise with the thumb in the canal, but this time the first finger grips the tragus (the anterior portion of the ear) instead of the ear lobe. Hold it, stretch it, rotate it, humming all this time at the proper pitch to vibrate the ear. About one minute of this should give good results.

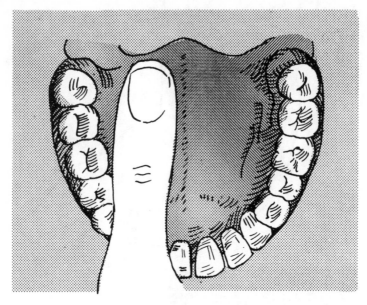

Fig. 12

YOUTH POSTURE WITH THUMB CONTACT ON THE ROOF
OF THE MOUTH, FOR REFLEX RELEASE IN MANY CON-
DITIONS

The hard palate is shown in figure 12. It is a vital area for stimulation. Either thumb fits perfectly here. The thumb from the same side has a soothing effect, while the opposite thumb has a stimulating reaction due to crossing over of the currents.

The body is in the same position as shown in figure 5, but now the contact is in the mouth. The cushion of the thumb is pressed upward on the hard palate on any sore spot found there, for many central reflexes in the head and in the body. The front of the palate reacts to the front of the body, the back portion to the back, and the center to the middle of the body, and each side reacts to that particular side. This makes it easy to localize reflexes. Being right under the brain, it is a positive pole with powerful reflex actions in its areas.

Most sensitive and responsive contacts are in the posterior portion of the hard palate. The stomach can be reached very quickly through this sensitive reflex area; also other abdominal organs will growl and show their response by the moving of gases. Energy currents which do not travel the usual path of nerve conduction are put to work in this way. Sympathetic reflexes are involved here, plus the wireless currents of energy flow which built the tracts and pipes of conduction in the first place by the soul's pattern in the embryonic state of the body. By gentle testing and pressing on these areas, reflexes will be discovered which reach every part of the body, benefiting eyes, ears, sinus areas, head congestion, etc.

This posture lends effectiveness to the contacts by using physical forces liberated in the body, through energy currents released and directed by the polarity of the hands and fingers through positive pole reflex areas in the head. Working with these reflexes and energies—research and discovery in application—makes one forget the posture taken.

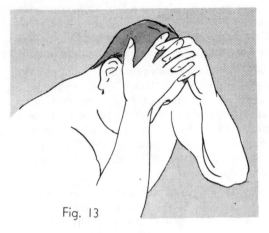

YOUTH POSTURE WITH THE HANDS
CLASPED OVER THE SIDES OF THE
HEAD ON TENDER AREAS, THE HEELS
OF THE HANDS PUSHING TOGETHER
AND UPWARD, FOR A POLARITY RE-
ACTION THRU THE PARIETAL BONES,
AND USED WITH HUMMING VIBRATIONS

Fig. 13

YOUTH POSTURE WITH HEAD-
MOLDING CONTACTS, THE
LEFT HAND ON THE LEFT
FOREHEAD AND THE RIGHT
HAND ON THE RIGHT OCCIP-
ITAL BONE ON THE BACK OF
THE HEAD.   FINGERS ARE
LOCKED FOR A GENTLE
SQUEEZING MOTION, UP-
WARD, BY BOTH HANDS, AND
USED WITH A HUMMING VI-
BRATION

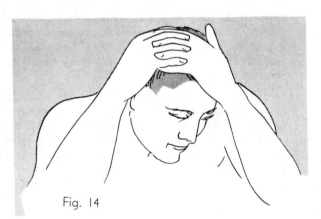

Fig. 14

The posture shown in figure 13 uses the same foundation while applying the polarity contacts to the head, placing one hand on any sore spot found and the opposite hand on the opposite side of the head. While in this posture, the parietal bones can be gently molded with the polarity contacts on each side of the head. *The fingers are locked,* which allows a *squeezing motion* to be made by the heels of the hands in an upward direction. This is in accordance with the dovetailed suture which gives with the breath. The idea is not really to move bones, but to give a stimulating or a soothing effect in the same direction in which the life currents flow and to augment the impulses by the polarity contacts and the influence of the posture currents applied locally through the hands.

The sides of the head reflex directly to the abdomen by one set of waves, and as a cross-over by another group thus constantly polarizing one side of the body with the other. Tissues and bones respond to polarity currents which hold them in position.

The gentle squeeze can be synchronized with the breath and with the humming pitch that vibrates these bones. Let each one test and prove these things for himself. This makes the effort original and interesting. We ought to discover deeper values and possibilities in ourselves every day.

Figure 14 presents a similar view as figure 13, but the hands are placed opposite each other, anteriorly on the forehead, and posteriorly on the occiput, diagonally across the head from one side to the other. Both positions of the hands are indicated here by merely reversing the contacts on the head. The molding effect and mild pressure is the same, as is also the humming and breathing in rhythm. These principles can be applied anywhere in the body with good results.

Vital Exercises with
Natural Breath Expression

The following exercises* (figures 15 through 23) use motion to integrate the Life Energy with the action, so the inside and the outside muscles both benefit in the effort. Five minutes of practice will convince anyone of their value.

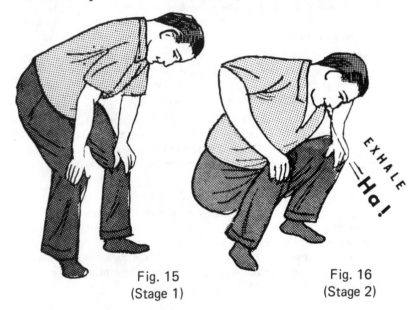

Fig. 15
(Stage 1)

Fig. 16
(Stage 2)

RELAX THE SHOULDERS AND FEEL IT BETWEEN THE BLADES AS A MOVEMENT. A fine exercise for the muscles of the shoulders, the abdomen, the thighs and the back. Useful in digestive disturbance, constipation, kidney inactivity and general sluggishness. Breathe out completely on going down (fig. 16) and breathe in on the rising (fig. 15). It is helpful to the brachial plexus by releasing the shoulders and neck tension. Let the head relax naturally forward.

---

*The rest of the exercises in this chapter were published in Dr. Stone's *Evolutionary Energy Charts* in 1960 and were specifically designated by Dr. Stone as a supplement to those published in his pamphlet *Easy Stretching Postures*. These exercises and those shown in Chapter 23 are an example of how he unceasingly continued to refine and develop his exercise practices for decades.

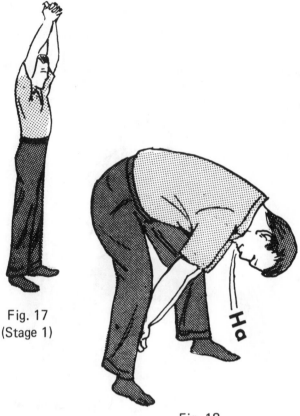

Fig. 17
(Stage 1)

Fig. 18
(Stage 2)

The above two-stage exercise is as natural as chopping wood* and so putting some real effort at the end of the stroke, which produces the natural sound of "Ha" at the end of the exhalation, as well as the elimination of the carbon dioxide, thereby completing the chemical action of the exercise—and all by natural means.

---

*This exercise is in fact referred to by many of Dr. Stone's students as the "Wood-chopper."

Vital Exercises for Toning the Body

The remaining exercises in this chapter are two powerful exercises using natural breath in the effort, which engages the inner Life Energy and most of the body muscles in one balanced expression of exhilaration of natural energy flow. The first exercise is illustrated on this page and the following page.

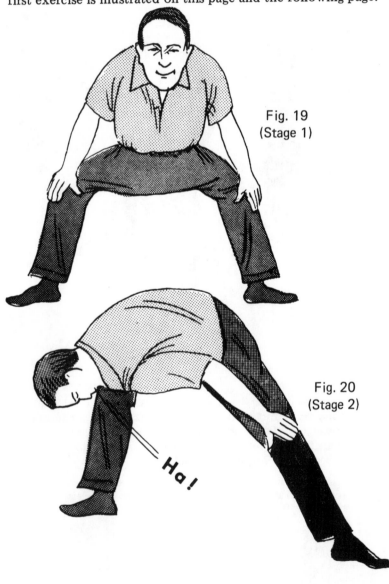

Fig. 19
(Stage 1)

Fig. 20
(Stage 2)

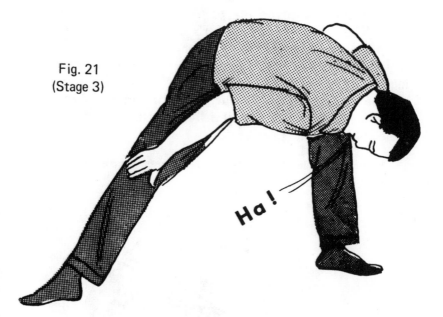

Fig. 21
(Stage 3)

Move from one side to the other alternately. Each time, exhale all the breath completely, with a loud "Ha" at the end of the movement, as the chest rests on the thigh.

Inhale naturally as you rise and change positions from left to right or right to left.

This exercise gives meaning and depth expression to our finer Energy Fields in the body, which need the exercise and resultant energizing of the otherwise stagnant currents even more than the muscular structure. But the muscles usually get all the attention, while the finer Energy Fields are neglected.

Exercise for Polarizing
the Energy Currents

The second exercise using the natural power of breath is the following—based on *the perfect neutral position of the body*. The embryo in the mother's womb is the beginning of the *perfect posture*, where all the energies can flow freely to build a perfect body.* To assist the body in repairs and building or rebuilding, some relationship to this primal position is used in many exercises for the particular purpose of *encouraging more Energy Flow*, especially when used together with the emphasis on the Life Breath.

This posture is wonderful for the relief of nervousness and excess gas.

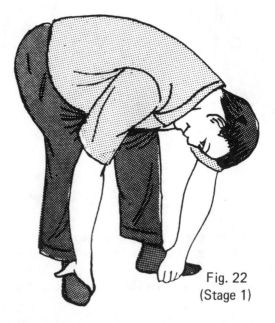

Fig. 22
(Stage 1)

---

*Dr. Stone's books *Energy* (in Volume I of the *Collected Works*) and *The Mysterious Sacrum* (in Volume II of the *Collected Works*) provide further explanation of this concept of the perfect posture for energy flow and human regeneration deriving from the embryo's position in the womb.

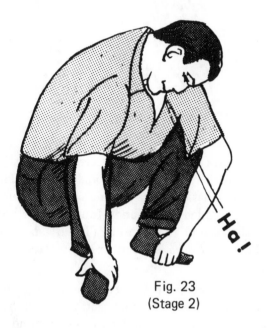

Fig. 23
(Stage 2)

This neutral position of the body is completed with the hands *under the arches of the feet,* so the Polarity Currents can be completed and flow freely. The elbow joints are over the knees, and the head is bent forward in a relaxed position in order to stretch the muscles of the neck and back.

Then a rocking motion is used—forwards and backwards—while the hands are pulling on the soles of the feet. Breathe out when the abdomen is squeezed by this motion, and breathe in when it is released. Next, rock from side to side and continue the same natural way of breathing as with the forward and backward motion. After that, rotate the body in a circular motion—clockwise and counter-clockwise—in as wide a circle as possible. This strengthens the pelvic muscles and is very helpful for lower back conditions.

23

Polarity Yoga for Health—Simple Stretches for All Ages

"The Infinite within is ever becoming."

The principle of *Yoga* is to join and balance the *tattwas*, or elemental functions of the five elements, with the *prana* energy, the breath of life, which animates them. The "Ha" of the sun's vital radiation principle and the "Tha" of the moon substance are blended in the body functions for health of the body as is the case in all of Nature. (The *Ha* and *Tha* combine to form the word *Hatha*, so familiar to Westerners from Hatha Yoga postures.)

Any posture or stretch in a *Yoga* designed for health must meet the requirements of the constitution of man by balancing "the above" (the subtle causal patterns of mind and sound current energy) with "the below" (the gross elements of solids and liquids in the structural frame). "As above, so below" is also mentioned in the ancient *Tablet of Hermes*. Tension fields in the five subtle elements of the body must be balanced in action and function, and united to the inner conscious center of "being". This is the object of *Polarity Yoga for Health* postures and practice.*

---

*The term "Polarity Yoga" and its principles and practices were published by Dr. Stone in 1970 in a small pamphlet titled *Energy Tracing Notes*, from which much of this chapter is excerpted. However, these ideas and the postures and exercises derived from these principles were simply a natural addition to and further development of Dr. Stone's Easy Stretching Postures. Dr. Stone personally explained and demonstrated Polarity Yoga with great enthusiasm in workshops in the early 1970s. And, although photos of Dr. Stone himself doing the exercises are available only for a few of the many variations he demonstrated in person, all of the exercises illustrated in this chapter are part of Polarity Yoga and/or the Easy Stretching Postures.

164

Prana is vibratory life; breath is the airy link with the liquids and solids in the tissue cells of the body. *Polarity Yoga* is a deeper stretch concept, for *conserving energy* by unification. It is more fundamental and corrective than any mechanical or physical exercise of muscles. And for time-saving and energy conservation it is a unique new application of Nature's constitutional energy and law of utilization.

The main objective is the release of subtle energy tension fields and stress blocks. Postural positions have their relationship to the mind patterns of the *tattwas*—and physiologically, through the connective tissue tension fields in the body. This release can be accomplished by special postures that put stress on the tension field in the connective tissue ligaments of the joints in the body, which are the cross-over points of energy flow in the structure. They are the hinges as well as the tendons that limit motion, and they are the cables of leverage in the body. The fixation lock of motion lies in the connective tissue as lesions of stress and pain produced by electromagnetic tension.

One of the special Polarity Yoga postures, personally demonstrated, also influences the duramater connective tissues that cover the brain and form the falx cerebri and the tentorium. They divide the brain into two lobes—the right and the left hemispheres—and separate the front (cerebrum) from the back (cerebellum) or hind brain and the constituents for motor function.

The meninges are three layers or covers of the spinal cord, which are extensions from the brain covers, with highly vital motor and sensory functions. The duramater is the outer connective tissue cover of these membranes that serves many purposes and is very important. It links the vertical lines of stress and movement with the horizontal lines of resistance in the five elements or *tattwas*. The duramater links "the above" with "the below" in the primary respiration process of life by co-ordinating the cranial bones' movements with the sacral motion.

The shoulders form the subtle airy level base in the physical body. The hip line center tension base is the water and earth level fulcrum base. In my Polarity Yoga for Health, *no artificial regulation of breathing* is necessary to obtain results. We are dealing with the *prana* distribution direct in its action on the five *tattwas* or elements in the body.

THE VISION AND ITS REFLECTION IN SPACE: The symbol of the cross in Nature's energy field is the vertical axis crossing the horizontal line of earth's energy. When the cross is folded up, it makes a perfect cube, the principle in balance of the two forces of the "superior" and the "inferior", as I have often illustrated. It is the Great Work of the soul when established and embodied in the consciousness, and it was called the "Magnum Opus" by Hermes in ancient times. It is "the spiritous earth" mentioned in his "Tablet". In the book of *Revelations,* it is described as the "City of Jerusalem", as a perfect square, descending from the heavens. This is one of the great secrets of the labors of the soul, opening the inner *chakras* or centers in the body and discovering the Life Energy behind the veil of matter. The Totem Pole of the American Indians conveyed the same message.

Practical application of this study of Nature's vital energy, as applied to the body for health and well-being, really has to be taught in person as an art of subtle energy stretches, with concentrated attention and devotion. Only five minutes of this practice every day can do wonders to keep the body fit. *But it must be done correctly,* so the energy flows, so the hinges and energy blocks are freed, and so the great "Masonic Arch"—the connection with the soul—is re-established consciously. This SELF-REALIZATION, by uniting and directing the energies inward, was the objective of the real temple builders of old.

Words and pictures cannot convey it nor can postures alone produce the maximum results. I am really surprised that even dedicated persons have to be shown this simple art over and over, again and again, to tune into the right octave of Nature's *prana,* the current of the Breath of Life, and the circulation of the cerebrospinal fluid as conductor for the life energy tissues. Then one feels the result of unobstructed energy currents flowing all over the body, as though it was tuned into the "Music of the Spheres". One feels so light, as if literally walking on air, similar in effect to a good POLARITY THERAPY TREATMENT. It is a real *release from tension* without drugs, without stimulation or instruments of any kind and without exertion. All that is needed is a fulcrum for a base, and the vision of the Creator's Love as the goal. These later research applications of fulcrum and leverage to the connective tissues add to the principles explained in earlier chapters of Part II and supplement the postures shown in Chapters 20, 21, and 22.

The feet are the basic fulcrum of the lowest level of precipitation, the emotionally chronic blocks in the water element of the body and also the earthy element of crystalization, inertia and solid waste blocks. Sore feet indicate the severity of these blocked conditions, preceding other illness. When the energy circuits cannot flow through the feet—the densest resistance furthest from the center of life's unconscious source and support at the solar (Sun) plexus—the circuit is then broken between the above and below strata (or planes) in the body, like a wheel off center.

The chart of the bottom of the feet is reproduced in this chapter to show the reflexes to the different levels or regions above, to which the circuits flow and upon which they react. This is accomplished when these foot-line areas are used as a *fulcrum base* pressure support, while taking these stretches of connective tissue *tension release* postures, with simultaneous shoulder-stretching.

The edge of a step on a stairway can serve as a fulcrum point if a good support for the hands to hold is available at the door frame or balustrade. The hand support can be about 16" ahead from the foot support, and 16" above it. If no such stairway is available, then it is easy to improvise by placing an 8" x 8" box, 32" long, or a long piece of wood at least 2½" high, in front of a door frame. One can then lean back while holding on to the door frame.

CHART
Nº. 4

FOUNDATION CIRCUITS

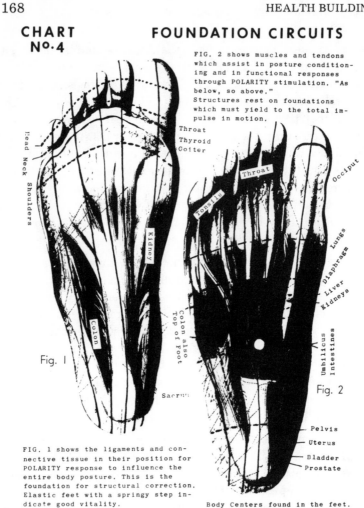

FIG. 2 shows muscles and tendons which assist in posture conditioning and in functional responses through POLARITY stimulation. "As below, so above."
Structures rest on foundations which must yield to the total impulse in motion.

Head Neck Shoulders

Kidney

Colon

Colon also Top of Foot

Fig. I

Sacrum

Throat
Thyroid
Goiter

Throat

Tonsils

Occiput

Lungs
Diaphragm
Liver
Kidneys

Umbilicus
Intestines

Fig. 2

Pelvis
Uterus
Bladder
Prostate

FIG. 1 shows the ligaments and connective tissue in their position for POLARITY response to influence the entire body posture. This is the foundation for structural correction. Elastic feet with a springy step indicate good vitality.

Body Centers found in the feet.

From Dr. Stone's book *Vitality Balance.*

Putting the fulcrum of support under the middle of the toes gives the greatest leverage release to the *NECK.*

Using the transverse arch (right under all the toe joints) as the fulcrum of support gives the *SHOULDER TENSION* the *most release.*

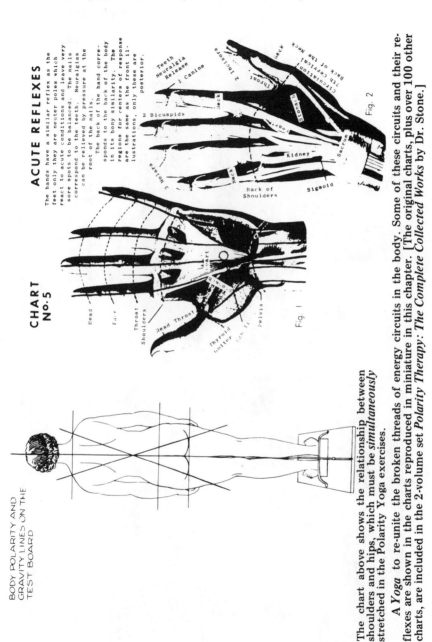

CHART No. 5

ACUTE REFLEXES

The hands have a similar reflex as the feet only they are neuter poles which react to acute conditions and leave very sore spots to be balanced. The nails correspond to the teeth. Neuralgias can be relieved by pressure at the root of the nails.

The back of the hand corresponds to the back of the body in its bony similarity. The regions for centers of response are the same as the front illustrations, only these are posterior.

Teeth
Neuralgia
Release

1 Canine

2 Bicuspids

3 Molars

Neck

Neck

Back of
Shoulders

Head

Face

Throat
Shoulders

Head Throat

Thyroid
Goiter

Pelvis

Fig. 1

2 Incisors

Throat

Neck

Circulation
7th Cervical
Back of the Neck

Neck

Stomach

Liver

Kidney

Sacral

Sigmoid

Fig. 2

BODY POLARITY AND
GRAVITY LINES ON THE
TEST BOARD

The chart above shows the relationship between shoulders and hips, which must be *simultaneously* stretched in the Polarity Yoga exercises.

A *Yoga* to re-unite the broken threads of energy circuits in the body. Some of these circuits and their reflexes are shown in the charts reproduced in miniature in this chapter. [The original charts, plus over 100 other charts, are included in the 2-volume set *Polarity Therapy: The Complete Collected Works by Dr. Stone.*]

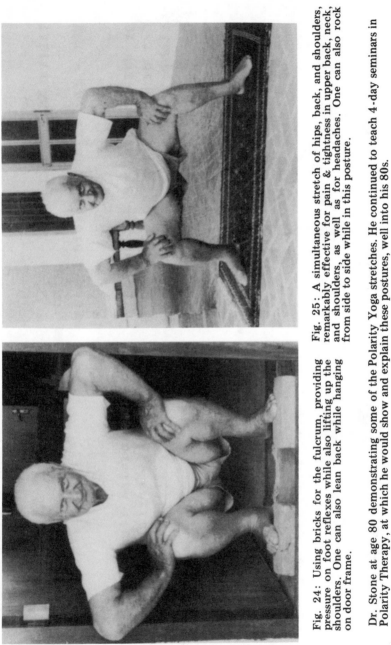

Fig. 24: Using bricks for the fulcrum, providing pressure on foot reflexes while also lifting up the shoulders. One can also lean back while hanging on door frame.

Fig. 25: A simultaneous stretch of hips, back, and shoulders, remarkably effective for pain & tightness in upper back, neck, and shoulders, as well as for headaches. One can also rock from side to side while in this posture.

Dr. Stone at age 80 demonstrating some of the Polarity Yoga stretches. He continued to teach 4-day seminars in Polarity Therapy, at which he would show and explain these postures, well into his 80s.

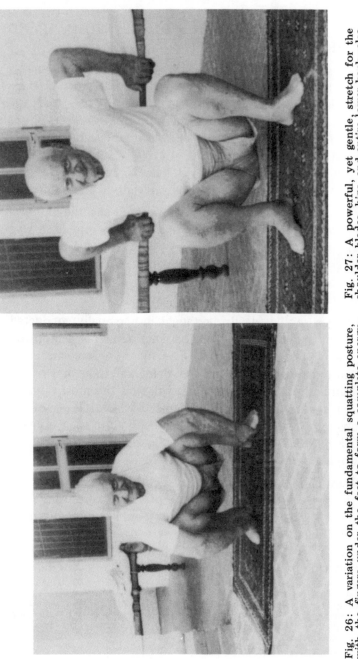

Fig. 27: A powerful, yet gentle, stretch for the shoulder blades, hips, and entire lower back—also activates digestive reflexes.

Fig. 26: A variation on the fundamental squatting posture, with the fingers under the feet to form a complete energy circuit. Extremely calming! One can rock back and forth, and from side to side gently while in this posture.

And just below the transverse arch, the STOMACH AND LIVER RESPONSE is obtained.

The sorest part on the foot level is the real lesion or energy block which needs help. Chart No. 4 from *Vitality Balance* (which is reproduced in this chapter in miniature) tells the story in the curved lines across the bottom of the feet. This is a new and specific application of *Polarity Yoga* fulcrum support and leverage for *Health*—RIGHT NOW, and all who have used it have benefited greatly by it. That is the Health-Building and maintaining Yoga, when rightly understood and practised.

Please note that the shoulder level base and the hip level base *must be engaged simultaneously in the one stretching posture* to move the *gross* energy blocks by means of the *subtle* energy in the united action on *both* levels. Unfortunately, many yoga postures practised today are not designed for the health needs of the students.

All this should ideally be taught in personally conducted classes and by doctors to their patients by actual demonstration,* and practised then and there by those who are interested in their own health and well-being and in helping others to attain and maintain it. Doctors will find this most valuable for themselves and for their patients, if they will personally demonstrate it to the patients and insist upon their doing it for *five minutes daily* as their part in the process of getting and staying well.

Many patients have come to me who were experts in Yoga as it is generally taught, and some of them were even Yoga Teachers; yet they had problems that could not be solved by all their Yoga practices, and they were greatly impressed and relieved by Polarity Yoga, as personally demonstrated to them. Acting by leverage application through opposite tension

---

*However, readers who are unable to consult a Polarity Therapy practitioner for such an in-person lesson can still benefit greatly by studying the illustrations and photos in this book and learning the exercises through experience.

fields, thus neutralizing and uniting them by extension and blending, is the alchemical process of TRUE YOGA FOR HEALTH, in the constitution of the body.

We cannot re-enter the womb of Nature and its neuter gestation field, but we can imitate Nature's process in overcoming resistance and energy blocks (or short circuits) by assuming neuter postures of embryonic life, which is always resilient and flexible. It is a path of life rather than of force; of rest rather than of conquest. This blending of the colorful varieties of energy lines and arches of beauty and stress in our temple-building is constructive maintenance and a true art of soulful expression. Our soul is really a treasure-house of the Lord's eternal gifts, more precious than pearls and emeralds.

Health-Building Yoga for the Infirm, the Aged & the Healthy
*More Gentle, Powerfully-Effective Tension Release Exercises**

In dealing with sick persons, an entirely different Yoga is needed to help their suffering through directing their Pranic Energies and establishing a balance in their subtle energy body, which is at war with itself and suffering just now. So, all exercises must be designed for that purpose: to establish health through the Prana flow, where it has been stopped through the resistance of too much grossness or by emotional disturbances which created blocks through mental upsets, fixations and false impressions.

The mind is the Neuter pole of the three Gunas. It is the Nucleus that governs the positive and the negative fields of the Pranas, the senses and the motion of the electromagnetic

---

*The rest of the text in this chapter is taken from an article Dr. Stone wrote for a South African newsletter in the 1970s, which was illustrated with photographs of many of his "Polarity Yoga" postures and exercises. Reprinted by permission of Mr. Sam Busa.

energy fields in the body. *Gentle guidance to redirect that energy into a balanced loving state is a most potent factor for health.* If this is coupled with exercises or postures to help control the negative mind impulses, as well as make the Prana Life Energy flow over the blocked areas in the body, seeming miracles can be accomplished. The secret lies in the simple conscious direction of the energies of the subtle body which does the feeling and acting.

This Health-Building Yoga is designed just for this purpose: to get well and stay well with just a few minutes of daily exercise even for the busiest person. It pays dividends in Health. The Principle involved is posture rather than strenuous exertion or accomplishment of difficult positions through exercise. The first objective is the release of the tension membranes of the body through relaxed postures, suspending the weight of the upper torso through the moveable support sockets of the shoulders.

The second objective is to free the lower portions of the body through the supports on the two hip sockets, which brings about a *complete repose*—a real neuter state of suspension like the embryo in the mother's womb. All things are possible in a neuter state, which is the only real isometric position of exercise. This is so subtle, gentle and deep that it is hard to describe on paper. It must be felt and done to actually get the benefit and to understand it. The approach and postures are unique and are designed for each individual's need, to assist the flow of their energy currents.

Health is the measure of man, not disease. There are over 1,500 "diseases", few of which are cured permanently. But there is only one life energy, which created all and supports all life and heals it, like the tree's life supports the trunk, branches, buds, leaves and fruits. The unit, the tree, the whole, needs attention more than the leaves and branches. It is the living current which supports all. Everything depends on it, in the life and well-being of that tree. It is the cause, while the details are the effects. Remove the cause of a disease and the effects will vanish. It is the disturbed energy in its flow which causes pains and disease symptoms. The electromagnetic forces are out of balance and must be restored.

By suspending the weight of the body on its natural supports, the tension membranes are stretched in the upper or lower portion of the body and relief is obtained at once. And then if you add the attention current of faith to this exercise, which uses the mind energy by attention and interest in the work, the results are marvellous. A little enthusiasm and cheerfulness destroys the gloom and depression immediately. *The mind must be employed with the exercise or posture*, so it is interesting, instructive and constructive for us. Mere mechanical, disinterested motion is useless, lifeless and gets little result, except wear on the poor body.

By hanging the head, neck and chest on the shoulder supports, the Brachial plexus is released of pressure and breathing is improved at once. The Pranas flow by the neck tension release. And the trapezius muscle is stretched. The hip sockets and their supports carry the total body weight. Relaxing in the squatting position while rocking in different directions and at various angles will release much pelvic tension and gases in the bowels. A little motion will employ different sets of muscles in this neuter posture. All our energy is freed to flow in this position, because it is nature's own design for creating a human being in the mother's womb. I illustrate this and give the whole Zodiac design in my books, based upon the four elements multiplied by the three Gunas (neuter, positive and negative), the three motions in all matter and space and energy fields. This is the one river, the etheric energy or the Tree of Life, which splits into four branches: the four elements of earth, water, fire and air.

NOTE: Some of the following postures and exercises are the same as or similar to those previously illustrated. However, a photo from a different angle can help clarify the posture. Also, many variations to each basic posture are possible, and some of those variations developed by Dr. Stone are depicted on the following pages.

The quickness and yet amazing effectiveness of these postures will be apparent only if they are tried *regularly* over a period of time. Once one is used to them and has achieved a comfortable routine, a full series can be done in less than five minutes.

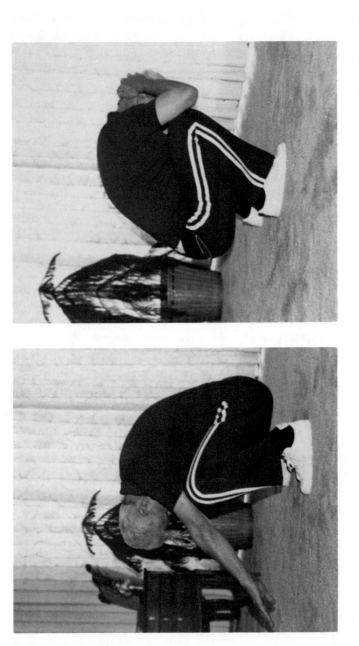

Figs. 28 & 29: Variations on basic squatting posture shown earlier. Gentle rocking back and forth, side to side, and in rotating circles can be done in both positions. Note that the downward pull on the head to stretch the spine must be slow and gentle. Note also that the feet should be *flat* on the floor, at least eventually after some days of practice.

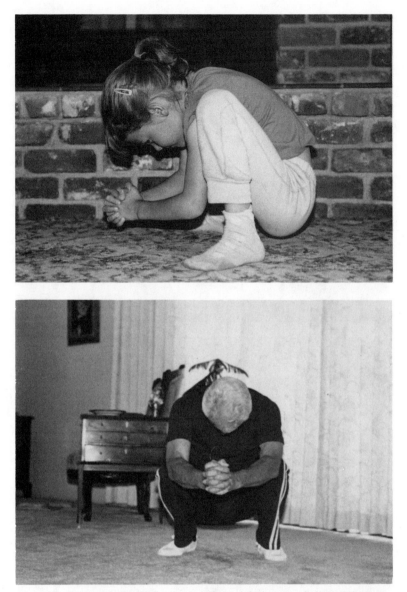

Figs. 30 (above) & 31 (below): Another variation on the squatting posture, clenching the fists and arm muscles periodically for an emotional
release, while also gently rocking. Let the head slowly drop down of its
own weight. Here we see how an easy, natural position for a 7-year-old
(fig. 30) can also be assumed quite easily by a man in his mid-sixties.

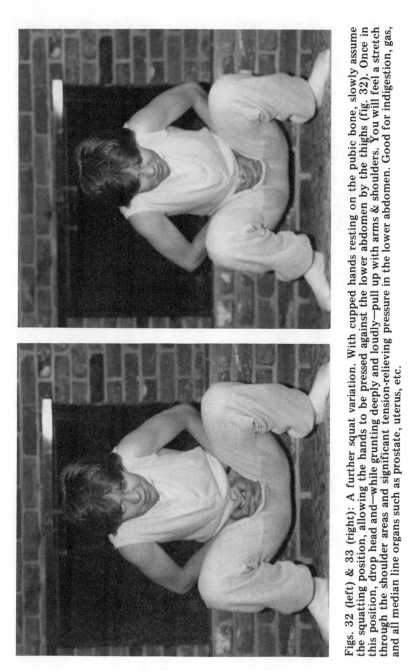

Figs. 32 (left) & 33 (right): A further squat variation. With cupped hands resting on the pubic bone, slowly assume the squatting position, allowing the hands to be pressed against the lower abdomen by the thighs (fig. 32). Once in this position, drop head and—while grunting deeply and loudly—pull up with arms & shoulders. You will feel a stretch through the shoulder areas and significant tension-relieving pressure in the lower abdomen. Good for indigestion, gas, and all median line organs such as prostate, uterus, etc.

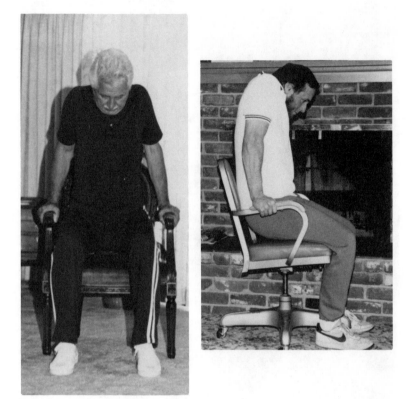

Fig. 34 (left) & 35 (right): A powerful exercise that can be done in almost any chair with arm rests. With straightened arms, the buttocks are lifted off the chair, while the head can lean forward and drop down into the shoulders, effecting deep stretches throughout the shoulders & shoulder blades. While in this position, one can also rock back and forth. Especially useful for the bedridden or crippled who cannot do most other exercises.

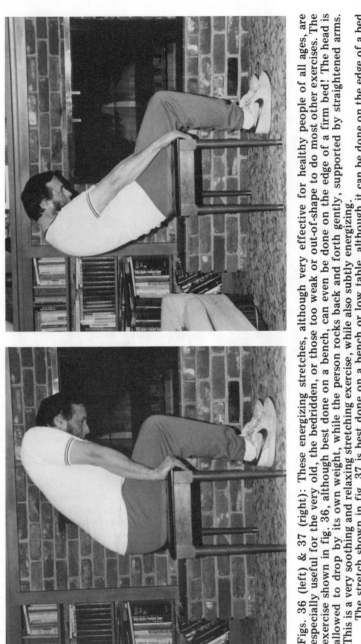

Figs. 36 (left) & 37 (right): These energizing stretches, although very effective for healthy people of all ages, are especially useful for the very old, the bedridden, or those too weak or out-of-shape to do most other exercises. The exercise shown in fig. 36, although best done on a bench, can even be done on the edge of a firm bed! The head is allowed to drop by its own weight, while the person rocks back and forth gently, supported by straightened arms. This is a very soothing and relaxing stretching exercise, while also subtly energizing.

The stretch shown in fig. 37 is best done on a bench or low table, although it can be done on the edge of a bed when the person cannot be moved elsewhere. Lean back with chin down and arms straight. Then pull while leaning back, raising the shoulders and stretching all the muscles along the spine very deeply. The feet remain flat on the floor during this stretch.

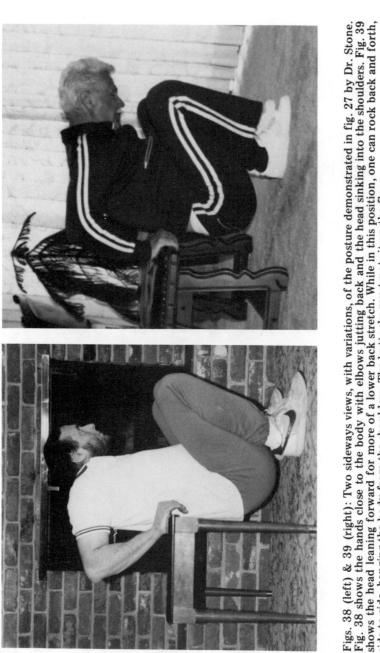

Figs. 38 (left) & 39 (right): Two sideways views, with variations, of the posture demonstrated in fig. 27 by Dr. Stone. Fig. 38 shows the hands close to the body with elbows jutting back and the head sinking into the shoulders. Fig. 39 shows the head leaning forward for more of a lower back stretch. While in this position, one can rock back and forth, side to side, hanging the body from the shoulders. The buttocks must not sit on the floor.

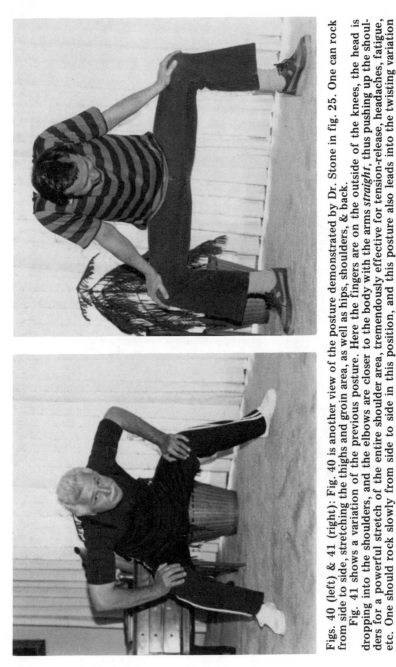

Figs. 40 (left) & 41 (right): Fig. 40 is another view of the posture demonstrated by Dr. Stone in fig. 25. One can rock from side to side, stretching the thighs and groin area, as well as hips, shoulders, & back.

Fig. 41 shows a variation of the previous posture. Here the fingers are on the outside of the knees, the head is dropping into the shoulders, and the elbows are closer to the body with the arms *straight*, thus pushing up the shoulders for a powerful stretch of the entire shoulder area, tremendously effective for tension-release, headaches, fatigue, etc. One should rock slowly from side to side in this position, and this posture also leads into the twisting variation shown next.

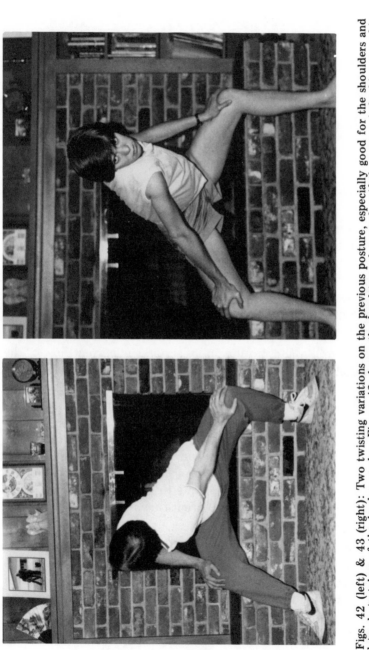

Figs. 42 (left) & 43 (right): Two twisting variations on the previous posture, especially good for the shoulders and lateral stretches of the back muscles. Figure 42 shows the head turned around as if the person is looking over his shoulder, while fig. 43 illustrates the twist while the head remains looking straight forward.

24

Energy Currents Control the Structure

"Life governs structure; structure limits life."

Life flows from within outward, and from above downward. The superior positive pole rules the inferior negative one by current flow. Disease is not an entity nor a fixed thing; it is nothing but a blockage of the currents of life in their flow and pattern circuits. Normal business and commerce has a similar flow—the exchange of goods and services. A depression, which is a serious disease in the business world, is nothing but a stoppage of the normal flow of exchange currents which carry the material goods wherever they are normally needed and used.

More life and motion, more action and current flow of the natural forces and paths of trade between the polarized elements constitute the answer to the problem. All the forces within man must be in constant communication and exchange with the universal forces outside in order to live. This is clearly demonstrated in the process of breathing. Stop that physiological exchange between man and the universe for a few minutes, and the whole process of life is interrupted. By whatever names we may describe the symptoms, calling them all kinds of "diseases", the current flow interruption is the real disease indeed.

Muscles and bones are part of the field which is the result of crystallized energy particles, deposited according to the pattern of the energy flow. The structure is the negative pole of matter and *must function as a field in harmony with the energy currents,* or the area is useless for proper function. Disharmony can be due to a positive locking of energy because of excess currents which cannot flow through, like in acute diseases with inflammations and congestions in the primary stages; or it can be due to a negative block expressed as flaccidity and inaction, as in chronic diseases where the energy block is complete and no real vital currents flow through with the exception of a trickle of stepped-down waves. By releasing the most negative pole in the triune fields, there is a possibility of re-establishing the current flow to some degree at least, even in chronic conditions.

Diseases are but symptom pictures of blocked positive or negative energy currents in the body, which cannot get back to the neuter pole which sustains them. Disease reflects the negative pole of waste deposits (solids, liquids or gases) and energy blocks in any area of the body. By working with living energy, the life force is represented in its positive aspects of polarity control impulses. Life responds to normal stimuli through energy currents and waves. It is our priceless heritage from the Creator. It is His pattern of things, used in the formation and molding stage in the beginning. Shall we use it, or bury its light under a bushel of theories and mental negations? *Effortless effort*, or doing by not doing it forcefully, is an old idea of the East, come to life again in our hemisphere. Working *with* life's currents is the whole idea in a nutshell!

Polarity operates in every field and function of the body. Corrections or remedies are effective only in proportion to how they act as balancing agents in these polarity fields and functions. The pelvis is the foundation of the body as the weight-bearing center of motion and action. It also has the unique function of preservation and perpetuation of the individual. Hence, it is of vital importance to maintain its polarity balance, so it can support the rest of the body and the integrity of the unit which depends upon its support—internally as impulse, and externally as gravity balance and the pivot center of motion.

The Easy Stretching Postures are based upon the finer currents of energy flow in the human body, promoting normal

*exchange between the universal supply currents and our indi-
vidual circuits.* Thus we tune in to the universal rivers of radiation and attract what we need for our daily existence. Such is
the law of life. We either obey it, or suffer sooner or later. A
simple lily in the field is arrayed in its natural beauty because
of its uninterrupted rhythmic energy supply, in tune with
nature.

Wisely using the body's own polarity is the key to unlocking blocked fields in the body without physical force or compulsion. Working with life's currents in the natural way, it does
the real work of normalizing energy flow through the body's
fields and re-establishing their circuits. Nature's way is gentle
and gradual in its process of construction and reconstruction.

The maximum benefit of these simple postures can be
obtained only by persons who are really interested, observant,
and will practise at least three to five minutes each day. Individuals engaged in strenuous mental or nerve-racking work
will find great release and rest after taking the two principal
postures and their variations.

When one cannot sleep at night and feels restless, it is the
airy principle in the body which is blocked and causes fear
and restlessness as a current interference; and, physiologically,
the cause is excessive gas and digestive disturbance. These
stretching postures will prove invaluable as a quick answer to
the problem, by establishing the flow of the downward current
at once.

These postures are also very helpful in emotional upsets,
because the current flow in the body is changed in a few
minutes. With the attention and interest added to the best
performance of the exercise, the change will be amazing and
very gratifying. When we forget our little self—the ego—
everything improves as by a magic touch. This also holds true
in extreme fatigue. Take the posture for a few minutes and
then rest a few minutes, and the recuperation will be faster
than ever before experienced. These posture stretches have

the polarity action of the constitutional currents of the body as a ready helper and mover of energy blocks.

We often hear about people in different parts of the world who can get more rest in one-half hour than we can in eight hours of sleep. The secret lies in activating and balancing the currents of the body, which do the work of recharging the fields or batteries of the body and keep it in good functioning condition. The human body is like an Aladdin's lamp. It has to be exercised or manipulated in the right direction, and placed so that the light and energy currents will fall where they are needed most. Polarity principles are the "Open Sesame" to the mysteries and functions of the wonderful human body, which is the shrine of the soul.

These easy stretching postures are the nearest approach to the position of the fetus in the mother's womb. In illness and severe abdominal pain, human beings automatically draw up their knees and quite unconsciously place the body in this ideal position, encouraging the wireless energy currents from Mother Nature to operate in repairing the body. My first book, *Energy: The Vital Polarity in the Healing Art,* contains a chart which graphically describes the position of the fetus in relation to the zodiac. As these currents work and the planets move, so does the fetus grow and develop.

This is mentioned simply to emphasize how natural and easy the postures are and how they activate the polarity fields for better current flow. Through these postures, the same forces which were at work building the body from the very beginning can continue today the wonderful work of repairing and maintaining the body. The results are increased vitality and a healthy glow and sparkle in the eyes, all of which naturally enhance beauty.

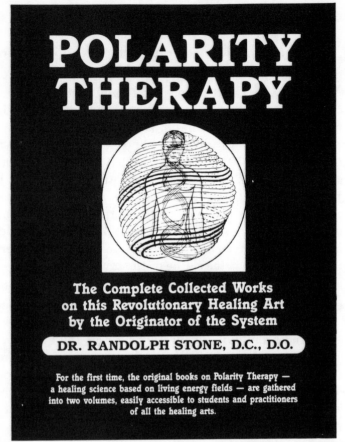

POLARITY THERAPY

The Complete Collected Works
on this Revolutionary Healing Art
by the Originator of the System

DR. RANDOLPH STONE, D.C., D.O.

For the first time, the original books on Polarity Therapy —
a healing science based on living energy fields — are gathered
into two volumes, easily accessible to students and practitioners
of all the healing arts.

This new collected edition comprises all of Dr. Stone's original works on Polarity Therapy. The contents of this two-volume set of large, *sewn-binding* paperback editions are as follows:

Volume I

Energy: The Vital Polarity in the Healing Art
The Wireless Anatomy of Man
Polarity Therapy

Volume II

The Mysterious Sacrum
Vitality Balance
25 Evolutionary Energy Charts
& various shorter works

For information on price or quantity discounts for schools, teachers, and health centers, please write to CRCS Publications (address on title page).

Dr. Stone's Polarity Therapy encompasses a wide variety of therapeutic techniques and theoretical considerations. Many types of therapeutic techniques and theories are currently being taught under the name of, or in association with, Polarity Therapy. The publisher urges the reader to contact the following two organizations, recognized by the Dr. Stone Trust, whose practitioners and training programs are directly based on Dr. Stone's work.

American Polarity Therapy Association
Statement of Purpose

The American Polarity Therapy Association is a non-profit corporation the purpose of which is:
1. To provide an organization for persons engaged in the study and practice of Polarity Therapy as described by Dr. Randolph Stone and to establish standards of competence and eligibility for membership which will confer recognized status upon accepted members.
2. To serve as a communication and support network for Polarity therapists, instructors, students, and any persons having interest in Polarity Therapy.
3. To establish and insure high professional standards for Polarity Therapists. Hence —
   a) To prescribe and uphold a code of ethics.
   b) To establish educational and training standards including required:
      1. curriculum
      2. number of hours of training and practice
      3. continued education
4. To develop the Association as a professional, responsible, ethical body and to insure that it is seen as such by other health professionals and by the general public.
5. To act as an information center, encouraging the availability of publications, media exchange, training, workshops, and conference announcements.
6. To function as a vehicle for research in the field of Polarity Therapy.

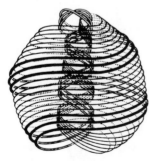

P.O. BOX 19459, SEATTLE, WASHINGTON 98109

Polarity Therapy Educational Trust
U.K.

PRACTITIONER TRAINING

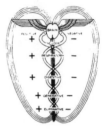

The Polarity Therapy Educational Trust provides a Three Year Professional Training in all aspects of Polarity Therapy. It also offers introductory seminars for the general public. The three year training commences every September. It is part-time, meets on weekends and includes a week's residential intensive in the second and third years. During the training, students learn both the theory and practice of Polarity Therapy. Dr Stone's texts are read in detail and students study both the subtle energy system and anatomical patterns of the body. Using this knowledge they learn to diagnose and correct imbalances in these systems. In this time students also experience their own self development as they apply the principles to their own lives.

Those interested in the Three Year Training should contact the Registrar at the address below.

The Polarity Therapy Educational Trust
c/o Franklyn Sills, Registrar
Broad Oaks, 69 Woodbury Avenue
Petersfield, Hampshire
GU32 2EB, U.K.

For a list of **qualified and**

registered practitioners write to:

The Polarity Therapy Association
c/o Jenny Harvey
11 Rowacres
Bath BA2 2LH
(0225) 26327